Antibacterial Drugs Today

W0193042

Antibacterial Drugs Today

A.P. Ball,* J.A. Gray[†] and J.McC. Murdoch[†]

* Department of Medicine (Sub-department of Communicable and Tropical Diseases)
The University of Birmingham, England
[†] Infectious Diseases Unit, City Hospital, Greenbank Drive, Edinburgh EH10 5SB, Scotland

MTP PRESS LIMITED *International Medical Publishers*

Antibacterial Drugs Today

Published in UK, Europe and Middle East
by MTP Press Limited
Falcon House
Lancaster
England

Second Edition
ISBN 978-0-85200-505-7   ISBN 978-94-011-8004-7 (eBook)
DOI 10.1007/978-94-011-8004-7

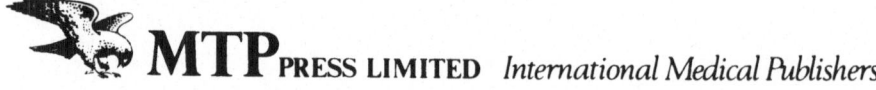

MTPPRESS LIMITED *International Medical Publishers*

© Copyright 1978 by ADIS Press
All rights reserved including that of translation into other languages. No part of this book
may be reproduced or transmitted in any form or by any means, electronic or mechanical, including photocopying, recording, or any information storage and retrieval system, without
permission in writing from ADIS Press.

Preface

Since the first edition there has been a great demand for this book. It has been revised to include up-to-date and new entries covering recent additions to the available drugs. As well there are now sections on clinical situations, or types of patient, presenting especial problems. The authors hope this new material will enhance the effectiveness of the book as a guide to this rapidly advancing and changing therapeutic situation.

A.P.B.
J.A.G.
J.McC.M.
July, 1978

Contents

Contents

1. Antibacterial Drugs Today

The basic concept of chemotherapy is the production of a drug which interferes with the growth, multiplication and survival of an infecting micro-organism, while at the same time producing little or no ill effects to the host. Since the development of the sulphonamides in the 1930s and subsequently, from the 1940s onwards of the antibiotics, there have been many drugs developed which are capable of exerting chemotherapeutic activity in a patient infected by a susceptible micro-organism (Kucers and Bennett, 1975).

It is important to remember that many infective processes are still not susceptible to a chemotherapeutic approach, and also that most febrile illnesses in children may be caused by an insusceptible infecting organism. Further, pyrexia can be due to diseases other than those caused by infection. The clinician must do his best to ascertain whether or not the febrile patient is suffering from infection by taking a very careful history and performing a full physical examination. Under ideal circumstances, where they are available, he will work in close collaboration with his laboratory colleagues, in particular, the medical microbiologist.

A great deal of time and effort in this field of therapy can be saved if the clinician and the laboratory worker are closely associated in the management of a susceptible infective process. While this book does not discuss in detail the type of specimen which should be taken from individual patients, it can be stated that unless a specimen is adequate and reaches the laboratory rapidly, the effort is wasted.

1.1 Mechanisms of Action

Chemotherapeutic drugs may either kill organisms: bactericidal action, or prevent multiplication: bacteriostatic action. In clinical practice this distinction is not as clear-cut as it is in a laboratory but in general terms, mixing bactericidal with bacteriostatic drugs is a bad therapeutic policy.

The action of the various drugs described in this volume, both from a bacteriological and pharmacokinetic point of view, is discussed under each individual group. In general the compounds may upset the formation of mucopeptides or directly affect the cell membrane, or they may interfere with protein synthesis within the bacterial cell itself. Mostly the exact action of chemotherapeutic drugs on organisms is not completely understood, but involves a very detailed knowledge of intracellular biology and biochemistry. The problems of synergism and the development of drug resistance by micro-organisms is another vast field of interest and the reader is referred to previous reviews on these subjects for further information (Hawking and Richmond, 1970).

1.2 Side Effects and Toxicity

Ehrlich's original concept of a chemotherapeutic agent which would kill organisms within the host without harming the host, has never fully materialised. As will be seen in the individual descriptions of the various antimicrobial drugs, none has escaped criticism on the grounds of significant side effects or toxicity. A vast literature on the subject has sprung up and this has been fully reviewed for antibiotic drugs by Manten (1972). The toxicity of the sulphonamides and other chemical agents, is referred to under the individual sections.

From a clinician's point of view, it is essential that a history of previous exposure to an antibacterial drug is obtained, and it is important not to expose the patient to the same, or a similar drug if there is even a doubtful history of side effects, allergy, or toxicity. Suitable alternative antibacterial drugs are almost always available, thus minimising the risks to the patient.

This book comprises, in the first part, concise descriptions of the important groups of antimicrobial agents with emphasis being placed on the more recently developed drugs. Sections 18 to 26 deal with particular types of organism, or groups of patients, which may be regarded as presenting the clinician with special problems.

2. The Sulphonamides

The sulphonamides and their antibacterial activity have been recognised since 1932 and have been in clinical use since 1935. The original sulphonamide has become the parent compound of a family of synthetic drugs, mostly with antibacterial activity, but some with hypoglycaemic or diuretic properties. The antibacterial sulphonamides have been largely superseded by the antibiotics and by co-trimoxazole (trimethoprim-sulphamethoxazole compound) because of the emergence of sulphonamide resistance, toxicity and greater *in vitro* and *in vivo* efficacy of the alternatives.

2.1 Antibacterial Activity

The sulphonamides, in the early years, had wide activity against both Gram-positive and Gram-negative bacteria. After nearly 30 years use considerable sulphonamide resistance has emerged and, in the Enterobacteriaceae has become common. Ball and Wallace (1974) in a study of urinary pathogens in a pyelonephritis unit showed that, by 1967, sensitivity to sulphonamides had dropped to 2% in *Escherichia coli* species and 4.5% in *Proteus mirabilis*. In 1972-73, after a fall in sulphonamide prescribing, the sensitivities had risen to 36.5% and 82% respectively.

Resistance is determined by degree of exposure and may occur during therapy. The majority of *Shigella* spp. and *Salmonella* spp. are resistant. Some staphylococci and streptococci are sensitive but enterococci are always resistant. Resistance in *Neisseriae* is common, gonococci having been reported as resistant in many cases since the 1940s. Meningococci have been reported resistant to sulphonamides, initially in America, but later in Britain. In Scotland in 1974, 52% of strains appeared at least partially resistant (Leading Article, 1974a). On the credit side, malarial and toxoplasma organisms, *Actinomyces* and *Nocardia* spp., and some *Chlamydiae* retain variable sensitivity.

2.2 Mode of Antibacterial Action

Sulphonamides exploit the difference in folic acid metabolism between man and his parasites. Whereas man absorbs preformed folate from the diet, bacteria and other parasites are required to synthesise folate from *p*-aminobenzoic acid (PABA). The sulphonamides sufficiently resemble PABA to act as false substrates, competitively blocking the enzyme dihydrofolic acid synthetase. The resulting effect on parasitic one carbon unit metabolism, secondary to folate deficiency, is bacteriostatic.

2.3 Pharmacology

Sulphonamides can be classified into three main groups:

1) Absorbable, rapidly excreted (short acting) e.g. sulphadiazine, sulphadimidine and sulphafurazole.

2) Absorbable, slowly excreted (long acting) e.g. sulphamethoxazole, sulphamethoxypyridazine, sulphaphenazole, sulphadimethoxine and ultra long acting compounds such as sulphametopyrazine, and sulphadoxine.

3) Non-absorbable e.g. sulphaguanidine and the succinyl and phthalyl sulphathiazoles.

With the exception of group 3, all sulphonamides are well absorbed orally and produce peak blood levels 2 to 3 hours after administration. Average blood levels for short acting members reach 50 to 100µg/ml. After absorption all are acetylated in the liver to a variable degree. The acetylated form is inactive as is the protein and red

cell bound fraction — the degree of which varies between individual sulphonamides.

The serum half-life of a typical short acting type, sulphadimidine, is approximately 2 to 3 hours. Short acting sulphonamides are rapidly excreted by glomerular
filtration and tubular secretion into the urine. Approximately 80% of the dose is
recovered in the urine, between 15 and 70% in the active non-acetylated form. The
long acting varieties are more highly protein bound and are subject to tubular reab-
sorption; consequently they have prolonged serum half-lives.

Parenteral administration results in rapid peak levels, but otherwise the pharmacokinetics resemble those seen with oral dosage. Sulphonamides penetrate poorly into
tissues, although cerebrospinal fluid levels range from 30 to 70% of a simultaneous
blood level. Biliary excretion is minimal.

2.4 Therapeutic Indications

Sulphonamides retain little place in the management of infective illness. In urinary tract infections, once a primary indication, many organisms are now highly resistant, although sulphonamides are still the drugs of choice in primary, uncomplicated
cystitis when the organism is sensitive. In meningococcal meningitis, resistance has
rendered sulphonamides of little use, and they are becoming decreasingly useful for
clearance of nasopharyngeal carriage states. Holten et al. (1969) have reported the
emergence of resistance after sulphonamide prophylaxis and recommend that their
use be discontinued.

It is doubtful whether any antibacterials, including the sulphonamides, are of
any benefit in non-invasive enteric illness, and if used in salmonellosis may encourage
a carriage state. Sulphonamides are of some benefit in nocardiosis, toxoplasmosis and
resistant malaria, but are probably best given in combination with trimethoprim (i.e.
as co-trimoxazole) for these conditions (see section 6). Prolonged treatment with
sulphonamides may prove beneficial in dermatitis herpetiformis, and sulphasalazine
may prevent relapse in ulcerative colitis. The mode of action of sulphasalazine in
ulcerative colitis is unknown.

2.5 Dosage

2.5.1 Short Acting Sulphonamides

Sulphadiazine, sulphadimidine and sulphafurazole are given orally in a dosage of
1g 6-hourly. In children, Kucers (1972) recommends a dosage schedule of 0.25g 6-
hourly up to 6 months, 0.5g 6-hourly up to 4 years, 0.5 to 0.75g 6-hourly up to 7
years and 0.75 to 1.0g 6-hourly from 7 to 12 years.

Parenteral administration is feasible but is extremely irritant. Sulphonamides should *never* be given intrathecally due to the risk of chemical arachnoiditis.

2.5.2 Long Acting Sulphonamides

A variety of these types are available with dosage intervals from 12 hours for sulphamethoxazole up to weekly for sulphamethopyrazine and sulphadoxine. The ultra long acting sulphonamides carry a high risk of hypersensitivity, including the Stevens-Johnson syndrome, and are best avoided. *especially in children.*

2.5.3 Non-absorbable Sulphonamides

Sulphaguanidine, succinylsulphathiazole and phthalylsulphathiazole are used in a dosage of 5 to 20g per day along with neomycin for the pre-operative suppression of bowel flora. The value of such preparations is not proven, but in view of the inactivity of these drugs against the anaerobes it seems unlikely to be beneficial.

2.6 Side Effects and Toxicity

2.6.1 Nephrotoxicity

The early sulphonamides with low solubility, sulphathiazole, sulphadiazine, sulphapyridine and sulphamerazine, tended to produce renal damage by precipitation in the renal tubule, resulting in haematuria, proteinuria, oliguria and even anuria. An element of hypersensitivity may also have been involved. However, renal toxicity is rare with later more soluble sulphonamides.

2.6.2 Haematological Abnormalities

These have been summarised by Murdoch (1965). Thrombocytopenia, granulocytopenia, haemolytic anaemia and fatal aplasia have all been recorded.

2.6.3 Pulmonary Disease

Pulmonary eosinophilia and generalised reactions with lung involvement and features of polyarteritis and the lupus syndrome have been reported with the sulphonamides (Leading Article, 1969). While fibrosing alveolitis has also occurred with the non-antibacterial sulphonamide sulphasalazine (used in the treatment of ulcerative colitis) there have been no reports of this reaction occurring with the antibacterial sulphonamides in current use, possibly because they are not derived from sulphapyridine as is sulphasalazine. Pulmonary eosinophilia, fibrosing alveolitis and bronchial asthmatic reaction due to sulphasalazine seem to be distinct from the rarer fibrosing alveolitis and apical pulmonary fibrosis recorded as complications of ulcerative colitis (Leading Article, 1974b). When sulphasalazine is withdrawn bronchopulmonary disease is usually reversed, but permanent lung damage or even death may follow. In all patients taking sulphasalazine symptoms of cough, weight loss and dyspnoea with radiographic signs should lead to a suspicion of toxicity due to this agent.

2.6.4 Hypersensitivity

Rashes and drug fever are not uncommon. Although Reeves (1975) found that sulfametopyrazine (a long acting agent) produced fewer side effects than sulphadimidine, the Stevens-Johnson syndrome, which may be fatal, is more common with long acting agents. Sulphonamides may account for up to 30% of cases (Beveridge et al., 1964). Carrol et al. (1966) reported a mortality of up to 25% in fully developed Stevens-Johnson syndrome, and suggested that the syndrome was commoner in children. It would therefore seem prudent to avoid sulphonamides of the long acting variety in this age group.

There is cross-allergenicity between the sulphonamides.

2.7 Drug Interactions

Sulphonamides are highly protein bound and may displace other drugs from binding sites, leading to subsequent toxicity of these drugs. Clinically appreciable interactions of this sort may occur with coumarin anticoagulants, and sulphonylureas. In addition sulphonamides may inhibit the enzymes responsible for the breakdown of coumarins and sulphonylureas with consequent risk of bleeding or hypoglycaemia. Enzyme inhibition by sulphonamide drugs may also result in increased serum levels of phenytoin and resultant ataxia.

3. The Natural Penicillins — Benzylpenicillin (Penicillin G) and Phenoxymethylpenicillin (Penicillin V)

The two so-called natural penicillins are both produced biosynthetically from *Penicillium chrysogenum* by fermentation. Benzylpenicillin (penicillin G) is formed if phenylacetic acid is added to the culture medium and phenoxymethylpenicillin (penicillin V) is formed when phenoxyacetic acid is added. Deacylation of penicillin G is brought about by amidase enzymes of bacterial origin which split off the side chain leaving the 'penicillin nucleus' or 6-aminopenicillanic acid (6-APA). The 'new' or semi-synthetic penicillins (section 4) are derived by grafting different side chains onto

6-APA so conferring widely differing pharmacological and antibacterial properties. The 6-APA nucleus itself consists of a thiazolidine ring fused to a β-lactam ring. This structure is converted into bacteriologically inert penicilloic acid by the enzyme β-lactamase or penicillinase which splits open the β-lactam ring (fig. 1). Some of the semi-synthetic penicillins possess bulky side chains which by stearic hindrance mechanisms protect the β-lactam ring from penicillinase; both of the natural penicillins and semi-synthetic penicillins such as ampicillin which possess less heavy side chains, remain entirely vulnerable to penicillinase action.

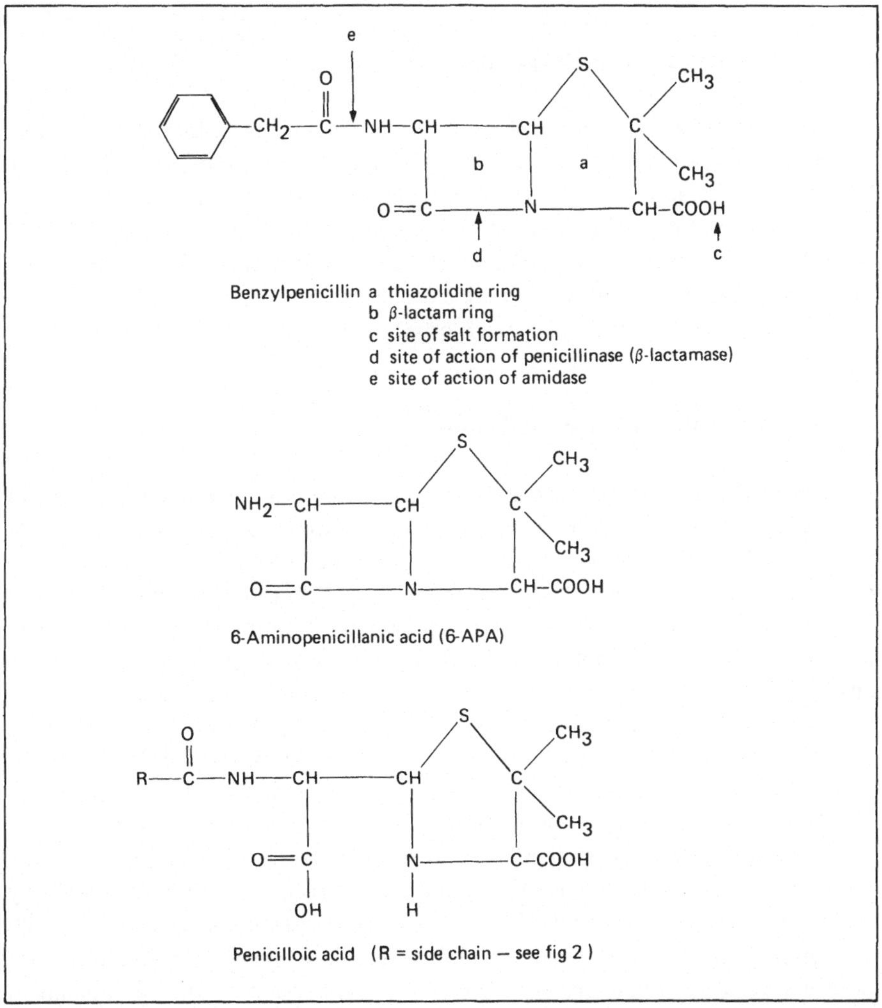

Benzylpenicillin a thiazolidine ring
           b β-lactam ring
           c site of salt formation
           d site of action of penicillinase (β-lactamase)
           e site of action of amidase

6-Aminopenicillanic acid (6-APA)

Penicilloic acid   (R = side chain — see fig 2)

Fig. 1. Structural formulae of benzylpenicillin, 6-aminopenicillanic acid (6-APA) and penicilloic acid.

The enormous disadvantage of penicillinase sensitive antibiotics may possibly be overcome in the future with the recent discovery of a β-lactamase inhibitor, clavulanic acid. This substance is produced from *Streptomyces clavuligerus* and is a β-lactam itself with some slight antibacterial action in its own right. Its important action, however, is that it has a strong affinity for β-lactamase and, combined in small amounts with penicillinase sensitive penicillins or cephalosporins, it may render them stable to enzyme destruction. Patient acceptability and freedom from toxicity have yet to be fully explored (Hamilton-Miller, 1977) but the prospect remains exciting.

3.1 Physicochemical Properties

After fermentation, penicillin is an unstable acid which can form a more stable but highly water soluble potassium or sodium salt. The potassium salt is known as 'crystalline' or 'soluble' penicillin which is an unsatisfactory term as it applies equally to any of the penicillins (Garrod et al., 1973). Penicillin G is unstable at low pH, and is quickly inactivated by gastric juice which generally precludes effective therapy by oral administration. Penicillin V, on the other hand, is not destroyed in the stomach and is quickly, though incompletely, absorbed in the upper small intestine.

3.2 Mode of Antibacterial Action

The penicillins, like the cephalosporins and cycloserine, interfere with bacterial cell wall synthesis. Disruption of the cell wall structure makes the bacterium unable to withstand variable osmotic pressures so that in the hypotonic solution of the environment it absorbs water, swells and bursts. During penicillin treatment there is an accumulation of peptides that would otherwise have been incorporated as cell wall precursors (Park and Strominger, 1957). Whereas cycloserine competes with its analogue D-alanine which is a substrate for the formation of the penta-peptide side chain of the cell wall backbone, the penicillins and cephalosporins act by preventing the cross linking of the glycopeptide backbone of the cell wall (Crofton, 1969). As bacterial cell walls contain mucopeptides not found in the host's cell walls, these antibiotics do not damage the cell walls of the host.

In normal growth bacterial cells are modified by the lysis of their inner walls by mucopeptidase enzymes and the remodelling and enlargement of their outer walls by synthesis of new protein. Spratt (1977) has reviewed the action of penicillin on bacilli and compared it with the action of mecillinam. The penicillins will bind onto any one of several penicillin binding proteins (PBP) on the bacterial cell, whereas mecillinam acts only at PBP_2. By interfering with the development of septa, the penicillins cause long filamentous bacterial forms to develop and as the antibacterial level rises higher, median bulges appear and finally cell lysis occurs with the release of the cell contents as a spheroplast (Spratt, 1977).

Low concentrations of penicillin do not interfere with protein synthesis and the cell continues to make mucopeptidases, so there may be a lag period of several hours before bacterial killing occurs. If the production of mucopeptidase is inhibited by the simultaneous administration of chloramphenicol, there may be no lysis of cell walls by penicillin. This may account for the antagonistic effect of chloramphenicol and penicillin when administered concomitantly (Crofton, 1969). Bactericidal drugs like penicillin act best during the growing phase of the bacteria and penicillin may be less effective when the cell metabolism has been slowed down by bacteriostatic drugs.

3.3 Antibacterial Activity

The natural penicillins remain the most effective antibiotics against sensitive Gram-positive bacteria and relatively the least toxic of antibiotics despite the many other antibacterial agents discovered since they were first introduced. Their antibacterial spectrum includes mainly Gram-positive organisms, the only Gram-negative species remaining mainly sensitive being *Neisseria meningitidis*, *N. catarrhalis* and some *N. gonorrhoeae*.

Gram-negative bacilli are almost all resistant to penicillins G and V with the exception of some *Bacteroides* spp. (Garrod et al., 1973).

3.3.1 Activity Against Streptococci

β-Haemolytic streptococci of Lancefield's Group A are highly sensitive to the natural penicillins which remain the drugs of choice in infections caused by these bacteria in non-penicillin-hypersensitive patients. Some strains of *Str. viridans* are very sensitive but many are now resistant suggesting that careful *in vitro* tube-dilution sensitivity testing is essential if penicillin alone is to be employed in the management of potentially life-threatening infections such as subacute bacterial endocarditis. Until recently there were no reports of resistance of *Str. pneumoniae* to the natural penicillins, but Hansman et al. (1971) have found some penicillin resistant pneumococci in New Guinea where prophylaxis against pneumonia was being given with monthly injections of procaine penicillin. *Str. faecalis* (enterococcus) is resistant to the natural penicillins.

3.3.2 Activity Against Staphylococci

When staphylococci are sensitive to penicillin the drug is still highly effective. Originally most strains of *Staphylococcus aureus* were fully sensitive (Barber and Rozwadowska-Dowzenko, 1948) but by 1961, particularly in hospital practice, almost all *Staph. aureus* strains were penicillinase producers (Morrison, 1961) and so highly resistant to penicillins G and V. Even amongst outpatients, the proportion of penicillin resistant staphylococci is considerable (Lynn, 1965).

The development of resistance to penicillin by staphylococci is not one of induction under therapy but one of substitution of non-penicillinase-producing strains by penicillinase producers (Barber, 1947; Barber and Rozwadowska-Dowzenko, 1948). The penicillin sensitive strains are eliminated by treatment leaving the penicillin-resistant strains to proliferate. Unfortunately, prior to the availability of penicillinase stable penicillins these penicillin-resistant strains were often extremely virulent and resistant to other antibiotics then available. *Staph. albus* may be pathogenic in situations where foreign materials such as synthetic heart valves, grafts and cerebrospinal fluid (CSF) shunts have been introduced into the body. It too, varies in its sensitivity to penicillin.

3.3.3 Activity Against Other Organisms

Penicillin G is usually effective against *Bacillus anthracis*, Clostridia, *Corynebacterium diphtheriae*, *Listeria monocytogenes* and the fungus *Actinomyces israelii*. *Treponema pallidum*, the causative agent of syphilis, remains penicillin sensitive.

Sensitivity testing is essential in assessing the likely response of the gonococcus to penicillins as a proportion of strains is now resistant. Both in South East Asia and in the USA strains with very high minimum inhibitory concentrations have been found and these require increasing doses of penicillin — often combined with pro-benecid — to give satisfactory therapeutic results (Leading Article, 1976). Even more disturbing is the finding of penicillinase producing gonococci almost simultaneously in the UK and USA for these strains are totally resistant to penicillin however high the dose is raised (Phillips, 1976; Ashford et al., 1976). Meningococci have until recently been regarded as highly sensitive to penicillin. A disturbing report from Athens (Contoyiannis and Adamopoulos, 1974) suggests, however, that some resistance may be developing.

3.4 Pharmacology

3.4.1 Penicillin G

In order to reach blood levels similar to those achieved with parenteral administration, 5 times the dose of penicillin G is required when the drug is given orally, even on an empty stomach. Hence penicillin G is seldom given by mouth. After intramuscular or intravenous injections of 600,000u penicillin G, high serum levels of up to 6 to 8µg/ml are reached within 30 minutes (Fishman and Hewitt,

1970). Diffusion into most tissues, including the fetus, is rapid but penetration of bone and CSF is negligible. However, the CSF antibiotic concentration rises to thera-peutically effective levels in meningitis when there is an increase in the extra-vascular compartment of intracranial tissue spaces. Penicillin levels in the CSF well in excess of the minimum inhibitory concentration (MIC) of invading meningococci and pneu-mococci are then easily obtained (Smith, 1972).

Probenecid has been used to delay renal excretion of penicillin. As it also inter-feres with the mechanism which transports penicillin back from the CSF to the blood (Fishman, 1964, 1966), it may have a theoretical added advantage in the treatment of meningitis with penicillin G. The bile concentration of penicillin is 2 to 5 times that in the serum but this is not of major therapeutic importance except possibly in the case of the semi-synthetic penicillin, ampicillin, whose antibacterial spectrum is more likely to include pathogens in the biliary system than are those of the natural penicillins.

The main disadvantage of both penicillin G and penicillin V is the very rapid renal tubular excretion. Antibiotic concentrations in the blood are very low at 4 hours and negligible at 6 hours after administration of standard doses. In order to obtain serum levels which are therapeutically effective after 6 hours, wastefully large doses of drug must be employed. Alternatives are to increase the frequency of administra-tion, to give the drug by continuous IV infusion, to combine these methods with an agent which interferes with renal excretion (i.e. probenecid), or to use one of the less soluble salts of penicillin G. Oral probenecid, 2g a day, in divided doses will enhance serum concentrations of penicillin several fold. Probenecid also competes with penicillin for protein binding sites in the blood, so releasing more penicillin in active form. About 50 % of the natural penicillin is protein bound in a loose form which may or may not interfere with its antibacterial effect (Rolinson, 1964; Kunin, 1967).

3.4.2 Benzathine and Procaine Salts of Penicillin G

Benzathine penicillin, one of the least soluble salts of penicillin G, gives lower but very prolonged blood levels which may last for one month after an injection of 1 to 2 mega units. Of intermediate solubility and duration of effect is the procaine salt of penicillin G which gives moderate blood concentrations for 12 to 24 hours.

3.4.3 Penicillin V

Phenoxymethylpenicillin (penicillin V) being acid stable survives gastric transit and is absorbed in the duodenum. Absorption is better in the fasting state and leads to high blood levels which in turn depend on the dose administered. Only about 35 to 40 % of the oral dose is found in the urine indicating that although absorption of penicillin V is much superior to that of penicillin G it is by no means complete. As with penicillin G, penicillin V is not significantly metabolised and it is rapidly excreted unchanged in the urine. The therapeutic level in the blood is low at 4 hours and negligible at 6 hours.

3.5 Therapeutic Indications

As a general principle the patient who is not hypersensitive to penicillin but who is infected with penicillin sensitive organisms, should be treated with penicillin. Its ready diffusability into all parts of the body (except bone and the non-inflamed meninges) is a great advantage. The dose may be safely raised to achieve high tissue concentrations without causing side effects or toxicity in most patients.

3.5.1 Streptococcal Infections

Infection with Lancefield's Group A β-haemolytic streptococci in the oropharynx, soft tissues or genital tract will respond dramatically to treatment with the natural penicillins. When fully sensitive, α-haemolytic streptococcal infections such as *Str. viridans* endocarditis should be treated for 4 to 6 weeks with benzylpenicillin followed by phenoxymethylpenicillin, assuming that peak blood levels of the latter can be shown to be in excess of the MIC of the organism isolated.

Str. pneumoniae infections such as lobar pneumonia or lung abscess should be treated with benzylpenicillin as the organism is very sensitive and the antibiotic will achieve high concentrations in the infected tissues.

3.5.2 Meningococcal Infections

Meningococcal septicaemia and meningitis can be effectively treated with penicillin G alone at present but the sensitivity of the organisms in the future should not be taken for granted. Because it so rapidly crosses the blood brain barrier when the meninges are inflamed there is no need to give penicillin intrathecally in normal circumstances.

3.5.3 Gonorrhoea

Gonorrhoea caused by strains which are fully sensitive will still respond dramatically to the natural penicillins which remain the drugs of choice. The MIC of strains of *Neisseria gonorrhoeae* in some parts of the world is now too high to rely on usual doses of soluble penicillin alone, particularly if sensitivity testing cannot be carried out, although single intramuscular doses of 5 mega units preceded by probenecid remain effective for most. β-Lactamase producing gonococci are of course totally resistant to penicillin and ampicillin. They are also resistant to streptomycin but remain sensitive to tetracycline, spectinomycin, kanamycin and co-trimoxazole (Leading Article, 1976).

3.5.4 Other Infections

Infections caused by penicillin sensitive staphylococci, whether *Staph. aureus* or *albus*, should be treated with the natural penicillins. Other infections for which penicillin G is the antibiotic of choice are syphilis, diphtheria, anthrax, erysipelas and infection with *Listeria monocytogenes*, bacteroides other than *B. fragilis*, and gas gangrene organisms.

Procaine penicillin is given daily by intramuscular injection in the management of syphilis. Benzathine penicillin by monthly intramuscular injection for prophylaxis after rheumatic fever is of particular use in patients who cannot be relied upon to take oral phenoxymethylpenicillin on a long term basis.

3.6 Dosage

3.6.1 Penicillin G

Benzylpenicillin, either as the potassium or sodium salt, is given either intravenously or intramuscularly in doses of 100,000 units or more. Depending on the sensitivity and site of infection, the standard adult dose of 250,000 units 4 to 6 hourly may be increased eight-fold or even more. When very high doses are employed, the intravenous route should be used and the potassium and sodium salts of penicillin should be alternated or mixed in an attempt to prevent neurotoxicity (Lerner et al., 1967; Brunner and Frick, 1968). Penicillin G is also available in tablet and lozenge form and as topical preparations. None of these is recommended.

3.6.2 Procaine and Benzathine Penicillin

Procaine penicillin should be given only by intramuscular injection, care being taken not to give an accidental intravenous injection. Dosage in non-gonococcal infections ranges from 300,000 to 1,200,000 units given once daily.

Benzathine penicillin is given by intramuscular injection in doses of 1,200,000 units once a month.

3.6.3 Penicillin V

Phenoxymethylpenicillin is given in tablet, capsule, or suspension form in doses of 250mg 4 to 6 hourly in adults.

Table I. In vitro activity of the various penicillins

Drug	Staphylococcus			Streptococcus				Gram-negative bacteria								
	Non-penicillinase producing	Penicillinase producing	Methicillin resistant	Grp. A	Grp. D	Str. viridans	Str. pneumoniae	Gonococci*, Meningococci	Esch. coli	Proteus mirabilis	Proteus vulgaris	H. influenzae	S. typhi	Kl. pneumoniae	Ps. aeruginosa
Benzylpenicillin (penicillin G)	+++	-	-	+++	++	+++	+++	+++	-	-	-	+	+	-	-
Phenoxymethyl penicillin (penicillin V)	+++	-	-	+++	+	+	+++	+++	-	-	-	+	-	-	-
Methicillin	++	++	++	-	+	-	+	+	-	-	-	-	-	-	-
Flucloxacillin	+++	+++	-	+++	++	+++	++	+++	-	-	-	-	-	-	-
Ampicillin	+++	-	-	+++	++	+++	++	+++	++	±	++	+++	++	-	-
Carbenicillin	+	-	-	++	±[1]	++	++	+++	±[1]	±[1]	+	+++	±[1]	-	±[1]

+++ High.
++ Medium.
+ Low.
± Variable.
±[1] Organism sensitive at high concentration.
- Resistant.

*Some strains sensitive only at very high concentrations. A very few strains totally resistant due to β-lactamase production.

3.7 Side Effects and Toxicity

Direct toxicity from the natural penicillins is rare.

3.7.1 Neurotoxicity

Very high levels of penicillin in the CSF may cause hyper-reflexia, coma, convulsion and myoclonus, the risk of which may be reduced by using a mixture of the sodium and potassium salts (Lerner et al., 1967). Large doses of the potassium salt should be avoided in patients with renal failure.

3.7.2 Nephritis

Nephritis is a rare complication of penicillin therapy and has been described in patients who have received very long courses in high dosage (Baldwin et al., 1968; Gilbert et al., 1970). Eosinophilia, rash, fever, haematuria and proteinuria are usual but not invariable features of nephritis. Dysuria, pyuria, eosinophilia and proteinuria without rash or fever were the presenting features in one case (Orchard and Rooker, 1974). It is not yet clear whether hypersensitivity alone or direct nephrotoxicity is the cause of the renal failure (Leading Article, 1974).

3.7.3 Haemolysis

During prolonged penicillin treatment red blood cells may be coated with an anti-penicillin IgG antibody giving rise to a haemolytic anaemia with a positive Coombs' test (Petz and Fudenberg, 1966; White et al., 1968).

3.7.4 Hypersensitivity

Allergic reactions occur in 5 to 10 % of those who are given penicillin according to Fishman and Hewitt (1970) who have described the problem in detail and reviewed the literature. They report that two types of reaction are noted clinically, immediate and delayed. *Immediate* reactions occur within 20 minutes of administration and vary in severity from pruritus and urticaria to laryngospasm, hypotension and death.

Anaphylaxis occurs in only 0.1 % of all penicillin reactions but is fatal in 10 to 25 % of instances; fatality is more common when the drug is given by injection. IgE is thought to be responsible for this (Type I) variety of reaction. A second type of immediate reaction may also occur between 20 minutes and 48 hours after administration. Manifestations of this type include fever, pruritus and urticaria, and although laryngospasm and hypotension do occasionally occur, fatality is uncommon. *Delayed* reactions take the form of skin rashes or serum-sickness-like illnesses and are the form most commonly seen. IgG and IgM are probably responsible for this (Type II) variety of reaction.

Nature of Penicillin Hypersensitivity

The exact nature of hypersensitivity is not yet understood but several different mechanisms are thought to operate and may account for the wide variety of clinical reactions encountered. Degradation products of penicillin include penicillenic acid, penicilloic acid and penicilloyl each of which may act as an allergen when combined with protein. Their antigenicity can be diminished by digestion with pronase which largely converts the potent polyvalent antigens to less immunogenic monovalent haptens (Munro, 1970; Shaltiel et al., 1971). Yet the removal or degradation of penicilloylated proteins does not completely stop penicillin allergies, some of which may be related to antigen polymer complexes which can form when solutions of penicillin are kept for a long time as in multiple dose vials (Fishman and Hewitt, 1970). Finally penicillin itself can act as a hapten antigen when bound to protein monovalently, or as a true allergen when more than one hapten molecule combines with the protein and reacts subsequently to form a network with polyvalent antibodies (Goslings, 1970).

Sensitisation to Penicillin

Penicillin allergy can occur in patients not previously treated with the drug. In such cases it is thought that the patients may have had prior exposure to the traces of penicillin so often present in milk, foodstuffs and vaccines. Alternatively, inhalation or skin contact may be sufficient to sensitise. Before giving a penicillin a careful history must always be taken of previous reactions to penicillins. With the exception of an

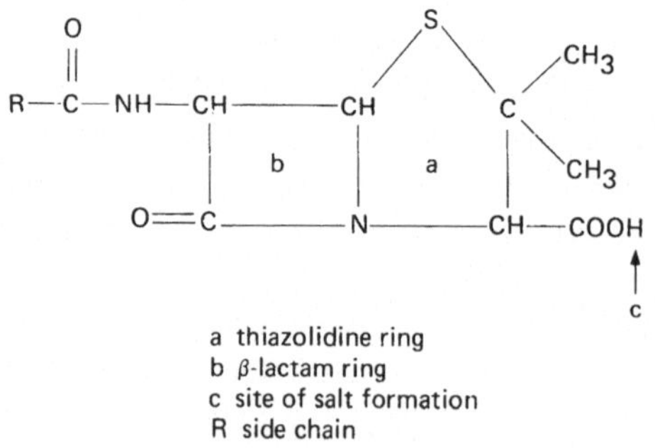

a thiazolidine ring
b β-lactam ring
c site of salt formation
R side chain

Fig. 2. Comparison of the structural formulae and properties of the various penicillins.

R	Generic name	Properties
$-CH_2-$ (benzyl)	Benzylpenicillin (penicillin G)	Narrow spectrum; acid labile; non-penicillinase-resistant
$-OCH_2-$	Phenoxymethylpenicillin (penicillin V)	Narrow spectrum; acid stable; non-penicillinase resistant
$-OCH-$ with CH_3	Phenethicillin	Narrow spectrum; acid stable; non-penicillinase resistant
OCH_3 ... OCH_3	Methicillin	Narrow spectrum; acid labile; penicillinase resistant
isoxazolyl ring with CH_3	Oxacillin	Narrow spectrum; acid stable; penicillinase resistant
(Cl*) Cl, isoxazolyl ring with CH_3	Cloxacillin (* dicloxacillin)	Narrow spectrum; acid stable; penicillinase resistant
F, Cl, isoxazolyl ring with CH_3	Flucloxacillin	Narrow spectrum; acid stable; penicillinase resistant
$-CH-$ with NH_2	Ampicillin (pivampicillin)	Broad spectrum; acid stable; non-penicillinase resistant
$OH-$ ... $-CH-$ with NH_2	Amoxycillin	Broad spectrum; acid stable; non-penicillinase resistant
$-CH-$ with NH_2 (cyclohexadienyl)	Epicillin	Broad spectrum; acid stable; non-penicillinase resistant
$-CH-$ with $COONa$	Carbenicillin	Active against G-ve bacilli; acid labile; non-penicillinase resistant

episode of delayed maculopapular eruption from ampicillin (see section 4.4.1), none of the penicillins should be given if a history of hypersensitivity is obtained and an alternative antibacterial should be used. Particular care should be exercised with atopic individuals.

Attempts to determine prior sensitisation by skin testing with penicillioyls or benzylpenicilloyl-polylysine are unsatisfactory and may actually induce sensitivity (Levine and Zolov, 1969) or even anaphylaxis (Ettinger and Kaye, 1964).

Recent animal experiments suggest that by combining the benzylpenicilloyl hapten with certain non-immunogenic carrier molecules not only is there a failure of antibody production but that specific immunological tolerance occurs. Translation of this experimental work in animals to man is still considered dangerous because of the risk of acute anaphylactic reactions (Leading Article, 1976).

Management of Immediate Hypersensitivity Reactions

Antihistamines, corticosteroids and adrenaline have been used with varying degrees of success in the management of immediate hypersensitivity to penicillin.

3.7.5 Side Effects of Penicillin V

Phenoxymethylpenicillin may cause any of the reactions described above for benzylpenicillin. It is usually well tolerated when given in standard dosage but may cause gastrointestinal upset in high dosage, especially when given on an empty stomach before meals in an attempt to promote absorption and increase blood levels.

4. The Semi-synthetic Penicillins

The separation of 6-APA from its side chain by amidase (fig. 1) has allowed a very wide variety of new side chains to be attached to the nucleus semi-synthetically giving rise to different therapeutic properties, including acid resistance as with the phenoxymethylpenicillins, penicillinase resistance as with methicillin and the isox-azolyl penicillins, and a wider antibacterial spectrum as with ampicillin, amoxycillin, epicillin, hetacillin and carbenicillin (fig. 2).

4.1 Phenoxypenicillins

Bond et al. (1963) studied the free and protein bound antibiotic concentrations in volunteers who had taken phenoxymethylpenicillin, phenethicillin and propicillin. In conjunction with the *in vitro* sensitivity pattern of these three drugs, they concluded that phenoxymethylpenicillin was the drug of choice for streptococcal infections, and phenethicillin for infections caused by non-penicillinase-producing staphylococci.

4.2 Penicillinase Resistant Penicillins

Certain bulky side-chains, when attached to the 6-APA nucleus can protect the β-lactam ring from the action of penicillinase. The first penicillinase resistant penicillin to be discovered was methicillin. This has the disadvantage of being acid labile, so that much of an oral dose is destroyed by gastric acid and the drug needs to be given parenterally to achieve good therapeutic results. The isoxazolyl penicillins, cloxacillin, oxacillin, dicloxacillin, flucloxacillin and the closely related nafcillin are resistant to both penicillinase and acid (section 4.2.2).

4.2.1 Methicillin

As the sodium salt, methicillin is readily soluble in water but is unstable in solution. It is quickly inactivated at pH levels below 2.0 (Rolinson et al., 1960). Methicillin is very active against staphylococci, both penicillinase and non-penicillinase producers, but it is less effective against other penicillinase producing bacteria. It is also active against other Gram-positive cocci (except *Str. faecalis*), but rather less so than is benzylpenicillin which should still be regarded as the drug of choice when the organism is sensitive to it. Gram-negative bacilli are resistant to methicillin.

Methicillin was initially reserved for the management of severe penicillinase producing staphylococcal infections, but it has now been largely supplanted by cloxacillin for this purpose. Increasing resistance of penicillinase producing staphylococci has been shown since methicillin was first introduced in 1960 (Gilbert and Sanford, 1970; Garrod et al., 1973) and may be as high as 4.11% of *Staph. aureus* isolates (Parker and Hewitt, 1970), or 10% of *Staph. albus* isolates (Kjellander and Finland, 1963). Isolates of methicillin resistant staphylococci seem to be heterogeneous and only a small proportion of the cells in these cultures show resistance (Sutherland and Rolinson, 1964). As they grow more slowly than the sensitive strains they present a problem of laboratory detection (Gilbert and Sanford, 1970).

Methicillin must be given parenterally. Peak serum levels of about 10μg/ml are attained 30 minutes after a dose of 1g. As with benzylpenicillin, methicillin is excreted rapidly by the kidneys so that by 5 hours the serum concentration is very low. Concomitant administration of probenecid will raise the serum concentrations. Dangerously high serum levels may be attained in the presence of renal failure. Only about 40% of methicillin is protein bound which is less than half that exhibited by the isoxazolyl penicillins including cloxacillin.

Therapeutic Indications

For the management of severe infections due to penicillinase producing staphylococci, the choice is between methicillin and the isoxazolyl penicillins. Disadvantages of methicillin are that it must be given parenterally and that it may occasionally cause bone marrow depression (Levitt et al., 1964) or nephritis (Brauninger and Remington, 1968; Baldwin et al., 1968). The main advantage of methicillin is the greater availability of unbound antibiotic, 60% compared with only about 5% of the isoxazolyl penicillins.

Dosage

Methicillin should be given in doses of 1g 4-hourly by intramuscular injection in adults. An attempt should be made to achieve peak serum concentrations 2 to 4 times greater than the MIC of the organism when dangerous infections such as endocarditis are being treated.

Patients hypersensitive to benzylpenicillin are also sensitive to methicillin.

4.2.2 Isoxazolyl Penicillins

These compounds are as acid stable as phenoxymethylpenicillin and in addition are resistant to destruction by penicillinase. They include cloxacillin, oxacillin, dicloxacillin and flucloxacillin. Recent reports have suggested that certain isolates of *Staph. aureus* have become 'penicillin tolerant' because although inhibited by low levels of these drugs, they are not killed at therapeutic concentrations and may therefore not respond to the isoxazolyl penicillins in clinical practice. Lacey (1977) who has reviewed the subject is sceptical that the small proportion of staphylococci in an isolate that are regarded as 'penicillin tolerant' is responsible for therapeutic failure and he regards other mechanisms as of equal if not greater importance.

The isoxazolyl penicillins may be administered orally or parenterally. Absorption is hindered by food residues and they should therefore be given orally one hour before meals. Oxacillin is the least well absorbed and it suffers further disadvantages in comparison with the other three drugs in that it is rather more rapidly excreted, penicillinase producing staphylococci are slightly less sensitive to its action, and it is rather less active against streptococci and pneumococci. Flucloxacillin is particularly well absorbed, producing blood concentrations twice those of cloxacillin at all times up to four hours (Garrod et al., 1973). All the isoxazolyl penicillins are very highly protein bound (94 to 97%) as compared with methicillin (see section 4.2.1) which largely offsets their greater intrinsic anti-staphylococcal activity. Little is known of the penetration of these drugs into the CSF, although they have been reported to be effective in meningitis. They do appear to achieve satisfactory concentration in the pleural and synovial fluids (Marcy and Klein, 1970).

Therapeutic Indications and Dosage

In view of the above it is evident that there is little to choose between this group of antibiotics and methicillin with its rather lower anti-staphylococcal activity and lesser protein binding. They should be reserved for severe infections due to penicillinase producing staphylococci. When the staphylococcus is sensitive to benzylpenicillin however, the latter drug remains the most effective and should always be used in preference to the isoxazolyl penicillins or methicillin. With the exception of flucloxacillin, the standard adult dose of the isoxazolyl penicillins is 500mg 4 to 6 hourly orally or by injection; flucloxacillin is given orally in 250mg doses.

Side Effects and Toxicity

The isoxazolyl penicillins suffer from the same disadvantages as methicillin and the other penicillins with respect to toxicity, but hypersensitivity nephritis is less common than after prolonged methicillin therapy. A transient rise in serum alanine aminotransferase enzyme (SGPT) and overgrowth of Gram-negative organisms and fungi have been reported (Marcy and Klein, 1970).

4.3 Other Penicillinase Resistant Penicillins

Other penicillinase resistant penicillins include diphenicillin, nafcillin and quinacillin, all of which yield low serum levels due to either irregular and incomplete absorption (diphenicillin, quinacillin) or to rapid inactivation (nafcillin). Any clear advantages over methicillin and the isoxazolyl penicillins in clinical practice have yet to be demonstrated.

4.4 Broad Spectrum Penicillins

4.4.1 Ampicillin

Ampicillin, a semi-synthetic penicillin which is only slightly water soluble, is given orally in the form of the free acid or parenterally as the sodium salt. Apart from enterococci *(Str. faecalis)* and *Listeria monocytogenes*, both of which are very sensitive to ampicillin, it is less active than benzylpenicillin against Gram-positive species, but unlike the natural penicillins, methicillin and the isoxazolyl penicillins its spectrum includes many Gram-negative bacilli. However, it is not penicillinase stable and is ineffective against penicillinase producing organisms whether Gram-positive (e.g. staphylococci) or Gram-negative (e.g. certain *Proteus* and *Klebsiella* spp.). Salmonellae, shigellae, most strains of *Haemophilus influenzae* and some *Esch. coli*, *Proteus* and *Klebsiella* spp. are usually fully sensitive. In view of the use made of ampicillin in the treatment of *H. influenzae* meningitis it is, however, alarming to note the increasing resistance of this organism (Turk, 1974; Clymo and Harper, 1974; Schiffer et al., 1974). It appears that the resistance of *H. influenzae* is due to an R factor mediated β-lactamase (Leading Article, 1976). Pseudomonas organisms are always highly resistant to ampicillin.

Mean peak blood levels of 2.0 to 2.5µg/ml are achieved in adults two hours after an oral dose of 500mg, irrespective of food intake (Bear et al., 1970). Doubling the dose doubles the serum levels. A blood level of 5 to 8µg/ml is found one hour after intramuscular injection of 500mg and very high levels of shorter duration after intravenous injection. About 24% of ampicillin is protein bound (Bear et al., 1970).

Adequate penetration of the CSF can be achieved with parenteral doses of 150mg/kg body weight per day. Very high levels of ampicillin are found in the bile where concentrations are up to 30 times those in serum. About one-quarter to one-third of an oral dose and up to one-half of an intramuscular dose is recovered unchanged in the urine. Probenecid slows the renal excretion of ampicillin and enhances the blood levels.

Therapeutic Indications

Ampicillin is a very widely used antibiotic because of its broad antibacterial spectrum, its availability for oral or parenteral administration and its relative lack of toxicity. However, it is often prescribed for indications where other drugs are more suitable. Because of increasing resistance of *Esch. coli* species some of its usefulness in infections caused by this organism has been lost. As a general rule, ampicillin should never be employed as a substitute for benzylpenicillin or phenoxymethylpenicillin especially in streptococcal, pneumococcal, gonococcal or meningococcal infections or in illnesses caused by penicillin sensitive staphylococci, as it is much less effective than the natural penicillins against these organisms.

Enterococcal endocarditis, exacerbations of chronic bronchitis, sensitive urinary tract infections, otitis media in young children and salmonella bacteraemia — but not uncomplicated salmonella enteritis — are important indications for ampicillin (see table II). *H. influenzae* meningitis has been successfully treated with large doses of ampicillin but the recent emergence of resistant type B strains (Schiffer et al., 1974) suggests that chloramphenicol, which crosses the blood-brain barrier well, will again become the drug of choice.

Dosage

The standard adult dose for chronic bronchitis is 250mg 6-hourly by mouth and for urinary infections and acute exacerbations of chronic bronchitis 500mg 6-hourly by mouth. Very high doses of ampicillin, up to 12g daily, may be given intramuscularly or intravenously in septicaemia or enterococcal endocarditis where treatment may need to be continued for 4 to 6 weeks.

Ampicillin has been used in the treatment of typhoid and paratyphoid fever but in some countries, particularly those where these diseases are endemic, it is only considered an alternative to chloramphenicol and co-trimoxazole. Ampicillin in divided doses of 4g daily should be given parenterally (or alternatively some of this may be given orally) in typhoid and paratyphoid fever and treatment should continue for at least 2 weeks. In the carrier state, ampicillin is considered to be more effective than

Table II. Indications for which the penicillins are treatment of first choice

Benzylpenicillin alone or followed by phenoxymethylpenicillin	Flucloxacillin or cloxacillin	Ampicillin	Carbenicillin
1) Sore throat, scarlet fever, erysipelas and bacteraemia due to Group A β-haemolytic streptococci	1) Serious infections due to penicillinase-producing staphylococci (e.g. bacteraemia, endocarditis, pneumonia, major wound infections and meningitis)	1) Exacerbation of chronic bronchitis and bronchopneumonia unlikely to be due to staphylococci (for treatment and prophylaxis)	1) Serious infections with sensitive *Ps. aeruginosa*
2) Lobar pneumonia	2) Staphylococcal osteomyelitis only where lincomycin or clindamycin are unsuitable because of toxicity or otherwise contraindicated	2) Acute otitis media in young children	2) Serious infections with ampicillin resistant *Proteus* spp. In both these indications, carbenicillin may be preferred to gentamicin especially in the elderly or those with renal failure
3) Acute bronchitis and bronchopneumonia where *H. influenzae* and staphylococci are unlikely to be pathogens		3) Non-penicillinase producing *H. influenzae* meningitis when chloramphenicol unsuitable or contraindicated (e.g. in the premature baby)	
4) Acute otitis media in adults and older children		4) Urinary tract infections, but only with known sensitive organisms (treatment and prophylaxis)	
5) Subacute bacterial endocarditis due to α-haemolytic streptococci (possibly combined with streptomycin)		5) Typhoid and para-typhoid fever only where chloramphenicol and co-trimoxazole are contraindicated or unsuitable	
6) Infections due to non-penicillinase-producing staphylococci		6) Group D streptococcal bacteraemia and endocarditis	
7) Meningococcal and pneumococcal bacteraemia and meningitis; listeria meningitis			
8) Puerperal and genital tract sepsis due to streptococci			
9) Tetanus and gas-gangrene (with antitoxins)			
10) Anthrax			
11) Gonorrhoea (most strains)			
12) Syphilis (procaine penicillin)			
13) Diphtheria (with antitoxin)			
14) Actinomycosis			
15) Rat-bite fever			
16) Prophylaxis of rheumatic fever (penicillin V or benzathine penicillin)			

chloramphenicol (and equally effective as co-trimoxazole), and may be given in doses of 1 to 2g daily by mouth for 6 weeks or longer for this purpose. It is not advisable to treat non-invasive *Salmonella* infections with any antibiotic as this may encourage a carrier state to develop.

In the treatment of sensitive *H. influenzae* meningitis high blood concentrations of ampicillin are necessary to get across the blood-brain barrier and the recommended parenteral dose should not be less than 150mg/kg body weight per day. Early reduction of the dose or substitution of oral therapy should be resisted in view of the greater difficulty in achieving good CSF concentrations as the meninges become less inflamed.

Side Effects and Toxicity

Ampicillin shares with the natural penicillins the same problems of hypersensitivity to the 6-APA nucleus, but it is also very non-toxic. Delayed rashes of a maculopapular erythematous type are, however, very common and are thought to be due to either impurities in the manufacture or to some factor associated with the ampicillin side-chain. Purification of the drug reduces the rash incidence by 50% but it still occurs. It is especially common in the presence of glandular fever (Pullen et al., 1967) and other conditions where lymphoid tissue is exuberant (Cameron and Richmond, 1971). There are now many examples of the drug continuing to be used during the course of a rash or being subsequently re-employed at a later date without adverse effects. There are also reports of fearsome reactions following subsequent exposure to even a single dose of the drug. Patients should probably be advised not to have ampicillin again, but assuming the initial eruption was a typical ampicillin rash, other forms of penicillin may be subsequently prescribed (Collaborative Study Group, 1973).

Despite earlier reports of deafness amongst children treated with high intravenous doses of ampicillin (Hambleton and Davies, 1974), there now seems less firm evidence that ampicillin is to blame. Dahnsjo et al. (1976) were unable to attribute varying degrees of deafness found in 6 of 37 children treated for *H. influenzae* meningitis to the large intravenous doses of ampicillin given.

4.4.2 Amoxycillin

Amoxycillin is a penicillin closely related to ampicillin in its antibacterial spectrum but it is more active against *Str. faecalis* and *Salmonellae* than ampicillin (Neu, 1974). It is sensitive to the action of penicillinase. Being acid stable like ampicillin it can be given by mouth but results in peak blood levels which are double those of equal doses of ampicillin (Sutherland et al., 1972). This permits a standard adult dose regimen of 250mg 8-hourly. Absorption is not interfered with by meals. It is now also available for parenteral use by both intravenous and intramuscular routes. It penetrates sputum better than ampicillin (May and Ingold, 1974) and may become the preferred drug in acute exacerbations of chronic bronchitis. Unfortunately drug rashes and gastrointestinal upsets occur, as with ampicillin.

4.4.3 Epicillin

This is another ampicillin-like compound, for either oral or parenteral use, with a similar antibacterial spectrum. It is less well absorbed than amoxycillin. Skin rashes with epicillin may be less frequent than with ampicillin (Brogden and Avery, 1972).

4.4.4 Hetacillin, Pivampicillin and Talampicillin

These compounds have no antibacterial activity of their own but after absorption they are rapidly hydrolysed into ampicillin and acetone (hetacillin) or ampicillin and ester (pivampicillin and talampicillin). Dose for dose, orally, hetacillin gives the smaller amount of ampicillin so it offers no clinical advantages (The Medical Letter, 1971). Both pivampicillin and talampicillin, however, give higher blood and urine levels than ampicillin (Daehne et al., 1971; Clayton et al., 1974). The antibacterial spectrum is identical to that of ampicillin. Talampicillin causes less diarrhoea than ampicillin (Knudsen and Harding, 1975) so is to be preferred to pivampicillin which often causes gastrointestinal disturbances (Wilcox et al., 1973).

4.4.5 Carbenicillin

This semi-synthetic penicillin is unique in its activity against *Pseudomonas* organisms, indole-positive *Proteus* spp. and *Serratia* spp. However, it is less effective than ampicillin against most *Esch. coli*, *Klebsiella* spp. and staphylococci and is not active against penicillinase producing strains of *Pr. mirabilis*. The drug is acid labile and must be given by injection. Concentrations of 100µg/ml of serum can be achieved by intravenous dosage schedules, but even these high levels are insufficient to eradicate some resistant *Ps. aeruginosa* strains.

Therapeutic Indications and Dosage
A 1g dose intramuscularly will give a peak level of 25µg/ml in the serum at one hour and the level falls to 4µg/ml by 6 hours. In the treatment of septicaemia, 20 to 30g daily may be required by the intravenous route. Carbenicillin is excreted by the kidneys and probenecid will help to achieve higher blood levels. This drug should be reserved for serious infections and septicaemia due to *Ps. aeruginosa* species such as are found in patients with extensive burns or with obstructive uropathy (Heineman and Israel, 1972).

Side Effects and Toxicity

Neurotoxicity may occur with very high dosage regimens and may be partly attributable to the amount of sodium administered, each gram of carbenicillin having 4.7mEq of this ion (Hewitt and Winters, 1973). Hypersensitivity is as for the natural penicillins.

4.4.6 Carindacillin (Indanyl Carbenicillin)

Carindacillin is acid stable and well absorbed as such after oral administration. It is quickly hydrolysed into carbenicillin and indanol in the body. Oral doses of 500mg or 1g will achieve peak serum concentrations of 10μg/ml. Higher doses tend to cause diarrhoea and it is therefore not practical to attempt to obtain the same antibacterial activity with this drug as from intravenously administered disodium carbenicillin.

Carindacillin may find a place in the management of some *Pseudomonas* or *proteus* urinary infections which are not deemed to merit more strenuous antibacterial therapy (Leading Article, 1973; Swarz and Storari, 1974).

5. Mecillinam and Pivmecillinam

Mecillinam is a new antibiotic derived from the 6-aminopenicillanic acid (6-APA) nucleus and synthesised from penicillin G. However, it is not classed as a penicillin, the difference being in the substitution of an amidino group in the 6 position in the β-lactam ring. This chemical manipulation affords the drug interesting new properties which are strikingly different from those of the penicillins in antibacterial activity and mode of action. Unfortunately mecillinam shares with the penicillins — except those in the isoxazolyl group — the disadvantage of being broken down by β-lactamase. This leaves an open β-lactam ring and a bacteriologically inert substance. It also raises the possibility that the formation of a penicilloate can lead to hypersensitivity reactions (Leading Article, 1976). Pivmecillinam is the orally absorbed ester of mecillinam (fig. 3). An appraisal of mecillinam is given in the supplement of the Journal of Antimicrobial Chemotherapy (July, 1977).

5.1 Antibacterial Activity

The most noticeable difference first recognised between mecillinam on the one hand and the penicillins and cephalosporins on the other was their antibacterial spectra (Lund and Tybring, 1972). Whereas mecillinam is very active against some Gram-negative bacilli, but much less active against Gram-positive cocci, the reverse is true of the penicillins and cephalosporins. Although *H. influenzae*, some *Proteus* spp.,

Providencia, Pseudomonas, Serratia and anaerobes such as *Bacteroides* are insensitive, mecillinam is highly effective against other Gram-negative bacilli including *Shigellae, Salmonellae* and ampicillin resistant *Esch. coli* (Williams et al., 1976). The possibility of resistance to mecillinam developing, especially during prolonged courses of therapy, as in the management of Salmonella infections, cannot be excluded (Anderson, 1977).

5.2 Mode of Action

Although closely similar in chemical structure to the penicillins, mecillinam acts in a different way. Even at high concentrations it produces large osmotically stable round cells, rather than inhibiting cell division and causing filamentous forms and osmotically fragile spheroplasts as happens when bacilli are subjected to the other β-lactam antibiotics (Spratt, 1977). Whereas the penicillins and cephalosporins bind to several different penicillin binding proteins (PBPs), mecillinam has a single specific target site, PBP_2 (Spratt, 1977). One of the reasons put forward to explain the synergy of β-lactam antibiotics and mecillinam is that the large osmotically stable round cells created by mecillinam are exquisitely sensitive to the action of the other drugs.

5.3 Pharmacology

Orally administered mecillinam is not absorbed. Its pivaloyloxymethyl ester, pivmecillinam, is well absorbed from the gastrointestinal tract and is used as the oral

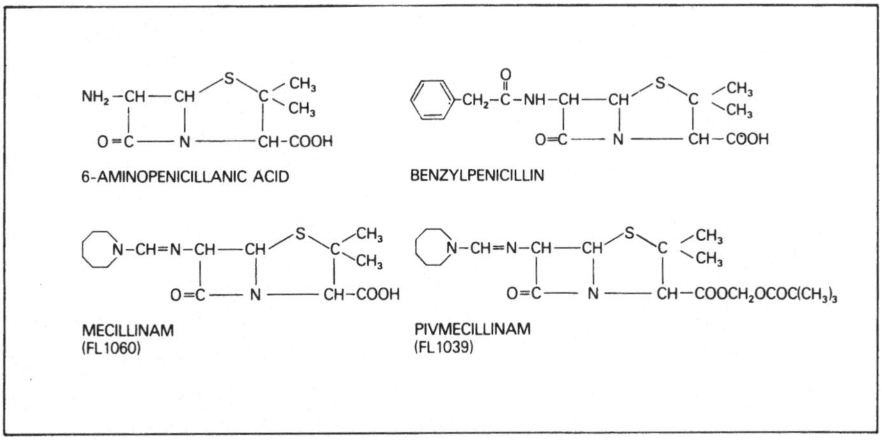

Fig. 3. Chemical structure of 6-aminopenicillanic acid, benzylpenicillin, mecillinam and pivmecillinam.

preparation. In itself pivmecillinam has no antibacterial activity but during or soon after absorption, it is hydrolysed into mecillinam.

In man peak serum levels of 6 and 12µg/ml were achieved respectively after intramuscular and intravenous injections of 200mg of mecillinam. After 400mg was administered by these 2 routes, peak serum levels were respectively 13 and 27µg/ml (Roholt, 1977). In human volunteers, Mitchard et al. (1977) found peak serum concentrations of between 6 and 9µg/ml after 200mg of intravenous mecillinam and 2µg/ml about 1 to 1.5 hours after the ingestion of 400mg of pivmecillinam. The absorption of pivmecillinam appears to be little affected by gastric contents. Urinary excretion is blocked by probenecid, leading to higher serum levels. Roholt (1977) showed that 45% of the administered dose was recovered in the urine in 6 hours without probenecid and 44% with probenecid. Biliary excretion also occurs (Clarke et al., 1976).

5.4 Indications

Although early clinical trials have been very favourable, it is too soon to assess the clinical efficacy of the drug, either by itself, or in combination with other β-lactam antibiotics with which mecillinam acts synergistically (Neu, 1977). As might be expected it has shown promise in the management of urinary tract infections (Verrier Jones and Asscher, 1975; Wise et al., 1977). Two studies suggested it was superior to amoxycillin and one that it was similar to co-trimoxazole in treating urinary infections and rather less likely to produce resistant strains (Bresky, 1977; Ishigami, 1977; Guttmann, 1977). More interestingly, mecillinam appears to be successful in treating acute typhoid and paratyphoid fever (Geddes and Clarke, 1977) and Salmonella carriers (Jonsson, 1977). In the latter situation the new drug vies with ampicillin and co-trimoxazole for pride of place. Pines et al. (1977) found combinations of mecillinam with amoxycillin superior to amoxycillin alone in managing purulent exacerbations of chronic bronchitis.

5.5 Dosage

Pivmecillinam is usually given in an adult dose of 400mg either 6 or 8 hourly. Intravenous mecillinam was used by Geddes and Clarke (1977) for the first 48 to 72 hours of treatment of patients with enteric fever, after which oral pivmecillinam was used to complete 14 days' therapy. Jonsson (1977) treated her Salmonella carriers initially with 0.3g pivmecillinam 4 times daily for 28 days, or, if this failed after 5 weeks, treatment was given with 1.2g pivmecillinam 4 times daily for 1 week.

5.6 Side Effects

Few side effects have been noted so far. Some skin rashes have been reported, occasional diarrhoea, sore throat and tongue with a sensation of 'chapped lips'. In 2 patients the SGOT and SGPT levels rose but no serious reactions have been encountered.

6. Co-trimoxazole (Trimethoprim-sulphamethoxazole)

Trimethoprim is a synthetic agent, related to the antimalarial drug pyrimethamine and was first described in 1962. Whilst retaining some antimalarial activity, trimethoprim has powerful antibacterial properties. This latter effect is due to blockade of bacterial folic acid synthesis, and a combination of trimethoprim with a sulphonamide has a strongly synergistic antibacterial effect. Trimethoprim is used in combination with sulphamethoxazole (SMZ) which has similar pharmacokinetic characteristics. The combination of TMP and SMZ in a ratio of 1:5 is known as co-trimoxazole.

Avery (1971) has extensively reviewed the earlier literature on co-trimoxazole.

6.1 Antibacterial Activity

The range of activity has been reviewed by Bushby (1973).

6.1.1 Gram-positive Bacteria

Staphylococci, streptococci (including pneumococci and enterococci) and *C. diphtheriae* are usually sensitive to co-trimoxazole.

6.1.2 Gram-negative Bacteria

The common Gram-negative bacteria, including *Esch. coli, Proteus* spp., *Klebsiella*, paracolons, *Shigella* spp. and *Salmonella* spp. are usually sensitive. May and Davies (1972) found 52% of *H. influenzae* strains isolated from the sputum of bronchitics to be resistant, but Williams and Andrews (1974) found all strains sensitive to co-trimoxazole. *Brucella* spp. are sensitive (Daikos et al., 1973), but *Neisseria* are less predictable. *Ps. aeruginosa* is almost always resistant, but Everett and Kishimoto (1973) found 75% of *Ps. pseudomallei* strains to be sensitive. The majority of strains of *Serratia marcescens* are sensitive (Gray et al., 1977). *Bacteroides fragilis* are moderately sensitive to the combination when the proportion of trimethoprim is increased (Phillips and Warren, 1974).

Rapid emergence of resistance to trimethoprim *in vitro* has been shown to be prevented by sulphamethoxazole, and sulphonamide resistant bacteria are frequently sensitive to the combination. R factor mediated resistance has been described by Fleming et al. (1972).

6.1.3 Miscellaneous

Mycobacteria, spirochaetes, mycoplasmas and chlamydiae are resistant, but malarial parasites are susceptible. Hughes et al. (1975) found co-trimoxazole to be effective in *Pneumocystis carinii* pneumonitis, but although Mossner (1969) reported successful treatment of toxoplasmosis, others have found no advantage in the combination (Feldman, 1973; Ruskin and Remington, 1976).

6.2 Mode of Action

Trimethoprim selectively inhibits dihydrofolic acid reductase and its effectiveness is therefore enhanced when the synthesis of dihydrofolic acid from *p*-aminobenzoic acid is blocked by a sulphonamide (fig. 4). This sequential blockade of the production of tetrahydrofolic acid is bactericidal (Hitchings, 1973). Trimethoprim binds to dihydrofolic acid reductase in bacteria with an affinity many thousands of times that in man (Burchall, 1973).

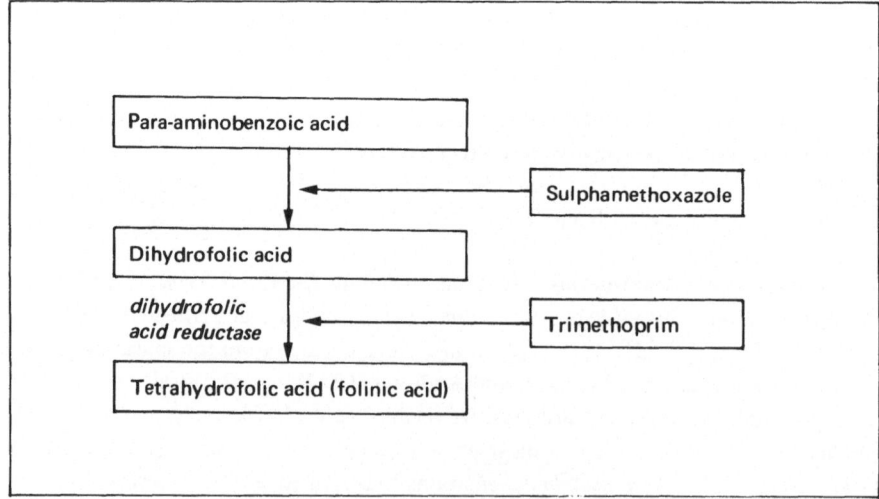

Fig. 4. Sequential inhibition of bacterial folate synthesis (simplified).

Sequential blockade of tetrahydrofolate production halts the synthesis of purines, pyrimidines and aminoacids. Then and Angehrn (1973) have shown that cell death in bacteria exposed to a combination of trimethoprim and a sulphonamide can be related to reduction in synthesis of thymine. Bushby (1973) has reported that the synergy of trimethoprim and sulphamethoxazole occurs over a wide range of ratios but is optimal at about 1:20 (TMP:SMZ). Synergy is sufficient to overcome bacterial resistance to one or other of the two constituents, but often only when concentrations are higher than those in the therapeutic range (Darrell et al., 1968). Synergy is maximal when the organisms are sensitive to both drugs.

6.3 Pharmacology

Schwartz and Ziegler (1969) have shown the combination is rapidly, predictably and almost completely absorbed from the gastrointestinal tract. Mean blood levels after a standard dosage of 160mg trimethoprim and 800mg sulphamethoxazole are: (a) 6 hours after the first dose: TMP, 1.10µg/ml; free SMZ, 20.3µg/ml; (b) In the steady state: TMP, 2.98µg/ml; free SMZ, 43.4µg/ml. Serum half-lives of TMP and SMZ are 14.5 and 11 hours respectively (Kaplan et al., 1973). This difference does not materially affect the blood levels in the steady state. Sulphamethoxazole is partly inactivated by acetylation and is 65% protein bound. Trimethoprim which has a wider distribution is 44% protein bound.

Both drugs are excreted via the kidney. Trimethoprim is excreted by glomerular filtration and excretion is maximal in an acid urine. Sulphamethoxazole is excreted by glomerular filtration and to a lesser extent by tubular secretion (Sharpstone, 1969) and its excretion is maximal in an alkaline urine. Welling et al. (1973) have shown that neither drug influences the excretion of the other and that renal clearance is reduced in renal failure. Kaplan et al. (1973) found that recovery of trimethoprim in urine amounted to 60% of the administered dose over 72 hours and that recovery of sulphamethoxazole averaged 85% (of which only 25% was present as free SMZ).

In renal failure, Sharpstone (1969) found that the clearance of sulphamethoxazole fell very little, short of oliguria, and Welling et al. (1973) showed the clearance of trimethoprim to be unaffected until creatinine clearance fell below 10ml/minute. The latter workers found that the half-lives of TMP and SMZ are increased 2-fold and 3-fold respectively in uraemic patients. The finding of deterioration in renal function in association with co-trimoxazole therapy (Kalowski et al., 1973) suggests that the combination should be used with utmost caution in patients with impaired renal function.

Therapeutically active levels have been found in human bile (Rieder, 1973), prostatic fluid (Meares, 1973) and in sputum (Hughes, 1973). Although concentrations of both drugs in the cerebrospinal fluid of healthy subjects are lower than in plasma, therapeutic levels are attainable in the presence of meningeal inflammation

Table III. Major indications for co-trimoxazole

Drug of first choice	Drug of secondary or alternative choice

1. *Urinary tract infections*
  a) Cystitis
  b) Pyelonephritis not requiring parenteral therapy
  c) Prostatitis
2. *Chest infections*
  a) Acute/chronic bronchitis
  b) Bronchopneumonia in chronic bronchitis
	1. *Salmonella infections*
	  a) Typhoid, paratyphoid
	  b) Invasive salmonellosis
	  c) Salmonella carrier state
	2. *Gonorrhoea*
	3. *Brucellosis*
	4. *Bacteroides infections*
	5. *Nocardiosis*
	6. *Melioidosis*
	7. *Toxoplasmosis*

Morzaria et al., 1969; Kirwan, 1974; Sabel and Brandberg, 1975). Absorption, metabolism and excretion of the combination in children (though not necessarily in neonates) appears to be similar to that in adults (Wilfert, 1973) [see section 21.4.3].

6.4 Indications

The major indications for co-trimoxazole are summarised in table III.

6.4.1 Urinary Tract Infections

Extensive experience has confirmed co-trimoxazole as a drug of first choice in this condition. Gruneberg and Kolbe (1969) obtained a cure rate of 92% in hospitalised patients, and Reeves et al. (1969) reported co-trimoxazole to be more effective than either ampicillin or sulphonamide alone. Similarly, Brumfitt and Pursell (1972) found significant advantages over ampicillin and cephalexin. Cattell et al. (1971), in adults, and Smellie et al. (1976), in children, have found long term, low dose, co-trimoxazole to be an effective prophylactic regimen in recurrent bacteriuria. Meares (1973) used the combination with success in acute prostatitis, and it has been used with some success in chronic prostatitis. However, resistance has appeared amongst urinary pathogens since the introduction of the drug, and Ball and Wallace (1974) found only 75% of *Esch. coli* strains isolated from women with recurrent bacteriuria to be sensitive.

6.4.2 Bacteraemic Syndromes

Darrell et al. (1968) and Bengtsson et al. (1974) have reported success in Gram-negative septicaemia, but more effective drug regimens will usually be available. Seligman et al. (1973) obtained indifferent results in endocarditis.

6.4.3 Gonorrhoea

Lawrence et al. (1973) found that a dose of four tablets (i.e. 320mg TMP; 1600mg SMZ) twice daily for 2 days resulted in a 98% cure rate in patients with gonorrhoea. Schofield et al. (1971) obtained similar results after a dose of two tablets twice daily for 5 days.

Co-trimoxazole is an effective agent in gonorrhoea and is suitable for use in patients who are sensitive to the penicillins and who can be relied upon to take the full course of treatment. It is ineffective against syphilis.

6.4.4 Chest Infections

Hughes (1973) found co-trimoxazole superior to ampicillin in bronchitics reducing sputum purulence in chest infections due to pneumococci and *H. influenzae*. True pneumonia also responded excellently.

6.4.5 Enteric Fever

Geddes et al. (1971) obtained satisfactory results in enteric fever using a dosage of 2 tablets 6-hourly for 14 days, and Kamat (1970) found co-trimoxazole superior to chloramphenicol. However, Scragg and Rubidge (1971) did not confirm the latter finding in children. In many areas chloramphenicol remains the drug of first choice, but increasing resistance in some countries indicates the need for an effective alternative. Gilman et al. (1975), reported co-trimoxazole to be more effective than amoxycillin against chloramphenicol sensitive strains causing human disease, but found little to choose between these agents if the organism was chloramphenicol resistant.

Limited success has been obtained using co-trimoxazole in the management of salmonella carriage states (Pichler et al., 1973).

6.4.6 Brucellosis

Daikos et al. (1973) treated 86 hospital patients with success in 78, and concluded that co-trimoxazole was effective in acute brucellosis, but that high initial doses (480mg TMP; 2400mg SMZ daily for the first 15 days) and prolonged administration (4 weeks) was necessary to prevent relapse.

6.4.7 Miscellaneous

Hanson and Woods (1975) have reported the successful use of trimethoprim and sulphadimidine in *Bacteroides* spp. septicaemia, but clindamycin and metronidazole are more effective alternatives. Co-trimoxazole is effective in nocardiosis and in melioidosis, and Hughes et al. (1975) successfully treated *Pneumocystis carinii* pneumonitis.

6.5 Dosage

Routine dosage in adults is 160mg trimethoprim and 800mg sulphamethoxazole which is contained in two proprietary tablets. This dose is given 12-hourly and produces blood levels in the optimal synergy range. In mild renal failure the same dosage may be used, but in severe failure (Ccr < 10ml/min) the dosage may need to be reduced. In children, Wilfert (1973) recommends a dosage of 200mg trimethoprim: 1000mg sulphamethoxazole/m² per 24 hours.

Co-trimoxazole is available as a parenteral preparation which requires dilution prior to intravenous infusion (refer to manufacturers literature for compatible diluents). Dosage is similar to that given orally, but may be doubled in seriously ill patients.

Dosage of co-trimoxazole in mild degrees of renal impairment remains the same as in other patients, but in those with moderate impairment the dosage should be reduced by 50% following an initial normal loading dose. Caution should be observed in severe renal failure (6.7.3) and an alternative agent may be more appropriate. Modification of the ratio of trimethoprim to sulphamethoxazole is not recommended in normal practice.

6.6 Contraindications

Co-trimoxazole should not be given in pregnancy or to neonates (see also section 21.4.3) or patients with a history of sulphonamide sensitivity, and should be used with care in patients with defective folate metabolism.

6.7 Side Effects and Toxicity

6.7.1 Haematological Abnormalities

The majority of interest surrounds the effect on human folate metabolism. This aspect has been reviewed by Herbert (1973) who concluded that co-trimoxazole should be used with extreme caution in patients who already have impaired folate metabolism due to folate deficiency. Such patients include pregnant women, alcoholics and those suffering from generalised malnutrition (e.g. elderly patients).

Animal studies by Udall (1969) demonstrated aplastic anaemia, neutropenia and thrombocytopenia, which were reversed by folinic acid. Kahn et al. (1968) had shown similar effects, due to interference with folate metabolism in man, although Whitman (1969) found only minor changes after doses of 1000mg of trimethoprim daily for a month. Since then, aplastic anaemia, neutropenia and thrombocytopenia have all been reported in man, but are infrequent, and may be related more to the sulphonamide moiety. Bateson et al. (1976) found co-trimoxazole to have no effect on serum folate in haematologically normal individuals, but Chanarin and England (1972), demonstrated a significant interference with response to haematinic therapy in patients with megaloblastic anaemias, in which conditions the drug is contraindicated. Hulme and Reeves (1971), suggested that acute neutropenia may be precipitated by co-trimoxazole in patients receiving immunosuppressives such as azathioprine, but Hall (1974) found that co-trimoxazole and azathioprine caused no significant increase in neutropenia when compared with azathioprine alone.

6.7.2 Hypersensitivity

Sulphonamide hypersensitivity has been previously described (section 2.6.4) and may be encountered occasionally in patients receiving co-trimoxazole. Skin rashes have been reported in patients receiving trimethoprim alone (Brumfitt and Pursell, 1972).

6.7.3 Nephrotoxicity

Deterioration in renal function, apparently due to acute tubular damage, has been described in 16 patients (Kalowski et al., 1973). Two of these had previously normal renal function, the other 14 having moderate to severe pre-existing renal impairment. The deterioration was reversible in only 13 of the patients. This finding led to a recommendation that co-trimoxazole should be avoided in renal failure. However, Tasker et al. (1975), studied 20 patients with renal failure on treatment with this drug, and found no evidence of drug induced deterioration. They concluded that co-trimoxazole may be used in renal failure subject to adjustment of the dosage.

6.8 Drug Interactions

Interactions with the sulphonamide component and other drugs may occur as previously described (section 2.7).

7. Chloramphenicol

Chloramphenicol was originally derived from *Streptomyces venezuelae* in 1947 and has been chemically synthesised since then. The literature on this drug has been reviewed by Kucers (1972).

7.1 Therapeutic Indications

Chloramphenicol initially enjoyed wide use, but it is now well known to be the cause of serious and often fatal bone marrow aplasia. Some clinicians believe that chloramphenicol should no longer be employed for the treatment of any disease process whatsoever. This extreme view is not, however, wholly acceptable throughout the world. Nevertheless, it can now be stated that the use of chloramphenicol should be restricted to the treatment of only a few infections, particularly fulminating enteric fever caused by either *Salmonella typhi* or *Salmonella paratyphi*.

7.1.1 Enteric Fever

There is no doubt that the clinical response to chloramphenicol in the enteric fevers is prompt and satisfactory, and compares favourably with the more delayed clinical response to either ampicillin or co-trimoxazole as alternative forms of treatment. In Southeast Asia however, chloramphenicol resistance — R factor related — has been found to be of importance, and workers in Thailand have noted a poor therapeutic response in typhoid patients treated with chloramphenicol (Lampe et al., 1974).

Lately there have been reports of resistance to chloramphenicol in *Salmonella* spp. in the United States, despite very little recent usage of the drug. The important clinical point found, was the rapid acquisition of resistance to chloramphenicol by salmonella during treatment, which in any event is open to question as the drug of first choice (Cherubin et al., 1977).

7.1.2 Other Indications

Controversy still persists as to whether chloramphenicol should be used at all, even for the treatment of enteric fevers. Nevertheless, it must be stated that many millions of patients have received chloramphenicol with benefit since 1947 and it would be unfair to condemn the drug outright.

A possible indication for its use is *Klebsiella pneumoniae* infection, although alternatives exist in the form of co-trimoxazole, injectible cephalosporins or kanamycin. There is no doubt also that chloramphenicol can be a useful alternative to ampicillin in the management of *Haemophilus influenzae* meningitis in young children. Ampicillin-resistant strains of *H. influenzae* have been isolated from sputum, and also from patients with meningitis in a few instances. The emergence of resistance of this organism to ampicillin suggests in fact that chloramphenicol may once again become the drug of choice in this condition.

Chloramphenicol should never be used in the treatment of infections susceptible to other less toxic antibiotics, and repeated courses should be avoided, even when the drug is occasionally used for recurrent enteric fevers. The casual prescription of chloramphenicol to an undiagnosed febrile patient is to be thoroughly condemned (Murdoch, 1974).

Chloramphenicol combined with streptomycin is the best treatment for Friedlander's pneumonia which, however, is a rare pneumonic disease.

8. The Tetracyclines

Many tetracyclines with a similar chemical structure and virtually the same spectrum of antimicrobial activity have become available since their introduction in 1948. A vast literature on them has sprung up and a number of detailed accounts of the tetracyclines and their development have been published (Kucers, 1972; Garrod et al., 1973; Murdoch, 1974). The most commonly used members of the tetracycline group are: tetracycline itself (the parent compound), oxytetracycline, chlortetracycline, demeclocycline (demethylchlortetracycline), and in more recent years, lymecycline, rolitetracycline, methacycline, clomocycline (chlormethylencycline), doxycycline and minocycline. While there are some individual differences between the various agents, they can be considered as a group.

8.1 Antibacterial Activity

The mechanism of action of the tetracyclines is believed to be interference with bacterial protein synthesis, the stage affected being probably the formation of peptide linkages (Garrod et al., 1973). In concentrations that are likely to be obtained in the blood stream and tissues, the tetracyclines are bacteriostatic and not bactericidal.

8.1.1 Spectrum of Activity

The tetracyclines resemble each other in the wide range of their antibacterial activity, and the term 'broad-spectrum' was first coined in connection with this group of antibiotics. In fact their spectrum is the broadest known. Susceptible species include not only Gram-positive organisms which are sensitive to penicillin, but also Gram-negative organisms which are not, and in addition mycoplasmas, rickettsiae and *Chlamydia* (Garrod et al., 1973). They are also active against *Treponema pallidum* and other treponemata, and have some activity against *Entamoeba histolytica* and the tubercle bacillus. However, they have little activity against most strains of *Proteus* spp. and *Ps. aeruginosa*. The activity of minocycline is generally slightly greater than that of the other tetracycline analogues, and this compound is active against many strains of tetracycline resistant staphylococci, including some methicillin resistant strains (Minuth et al., 1974).

8.1.2 Development of Resistance

Most bacteria are slow to acquire resistance to the tetracyclines. Nevertheless, since their widespread and often indiscriminate use, resistant strains of staphylococci and various coliform bacilli have gradually become fairly common and this has lead to a decrease in their usefulness, especially in the hospital environment. Resistance in haemolytic streptococci and pneumococci has also occurred in recent years and some diminution in the sensitivity of strains of *H. influenzae* has been observed (Garrod et al., 1973).

There is generally complete cross resistance between most analogues, and an organism resistant to one tetracycline is usually equally resistant to any other. The only exception to this occurs with minocycline and strains of *Staph. aureus*.

8.2 Pharmacology

With the exception of rolitetracycline which is only given parenterally, all the commonly used tetracyclines *(vide supra)* may be given orally. Absorption occurs from all levels of the alimentary tract from the stomach onwards. With most analogues, absorption is increased and higher blood levels are attained if the drug is taken during the fasting state, but with doxycycline and minocycline absorption does not appear to be appreciably influenced by the presence of food. However, with all compounds absorption may be adversely affected by the presence of aluminium, calcium, magnesium or iron salts due to the formation of chelates.

Following absorption a proportion of the ingested dose is broken down in the liver by metabolic processes. Effective levels are achieved for up to 6 hours with tetracycline, oxytetracycline and chlortetracycline, but more prolonged levels are attained with demeclocycline, methacycline, minocycline and doxycycline which have longer serum half-lives. With doxycycline in particular, adequate serum levels may persist for up to 24 hours and this drug is given on a once-daily dosage regimen.

The tetracyclines diffuse well into most body fluids and tissues, but diffusion across the blood-brain barrier is poor — except when the meninges are inflamed. They are excreted in both the bile and the urine, and in the former concentrations may be up to 10 to 20 times those in the blood. In the presence of renal failure, doxycycline is the only tetracycline which can be safely administered, as the others — with the possible exception of minocycline — have been associated with clinical and biochemical evidence of further deterioration in renal function.

8.3 Therapeutic Indications

In sophisticated hospital environments there are now many organisms which are tetracycline resistant — including *Staph. aureus* and many Gram-negative organisms

Table IV. Major indications for the tetracyclines

Drug of first choice	Drug of secondary or alternative choice
1. Acute exacerbations of chronic bronchitis	1. Syphilis (in penicillin-sensitive patients)
2. Non-specific urethritis	2. Actinomycosis
3. Pneumonia due to *Mycoplasma pneumoniae;* Q-fever; psittacosis	3. Anthrax
4. Acne vulgaris (pustular)	
5. Brucellosis	
6. Lymphogranuloma venereum	
7. Trachoma	
8. Rickettsial infections	
9. Leptospirosis	
10. Typhus	

— and it can be said that at present the tetracyclines have little or no place in the management of infections acquired in hospital. While some resistant strains, particularly of *Staph. aureus,* may be fully sensitive to minocycline, the place of this drug in hospital practice has still to be fully evaluated.

Outside the hospital environment however, the tetracyclines may be used in a variety of infections (table IV). In chronic bronchitic patients the tetracyclines still have a place in the treatment of acute exacerbations. Similarly, they are still the drugs of first choice for pneumonia caused by *Mycoplasma pneumoniae,* and for psittacosis, non-specific urethritis, lymphogranuloma venereum, rickettsial infections, trachoma, brucellosis and acne vulgaris. In actinomycosis, anthrax and syphilis the tetracyclines also offer an alternative to penicillin. On the other hand, because of the emergence of tetracycline resistant strains of haemolytic streptococci and pneumococci over the years they should not be used in the primary treatment of sore throats or pneumococcal pneumonia. While there can be no doubt that the tetracyclines have been infinitely valuable in the management of many infections in past years, the indications for their use are diminishing, particularly in developed countries.

8.4 Side Effects and Toxicity

The most common side effect with oral tetracycline treatment is looseness of the stools. The exact cause of this is not known, but in some cases there is an overgrowth of *Candida albicans* leading to the oro-genital syndrome. Serious invasive candidiasis leading to death is fortunately rare, and staphylococcal entero-colitis is now much less common than it used to be in hospitals.

Other side effects occasionally observed include hypersensitivity reactions, skin reactions (including photosensitivity), pain at the injection site with parenteral administration and, on rare occasions, marrow dyscrasias. Dizziness has been a commonly reported side effect of minocycline.

8.4.1 Tooth Discoloration

The use of tetracycline during tooth development (i.e. during the last trimester of pregnancy, the neonatal period and early childhood) can lead to discoloration of teeth, although this phenomenon has generally only been seen in patients who have received large doses over a prolonged period. Oxytetracycline and doxycycline are said to induce less discoloration than most of the other analogues (see section 21.4.5).

8.4.2 Renal Toxicity

In general, the tetracyclines should not be given to patients with renal failure as they may cause clinical and biochemical evidence of deterioration in renal function. A possible exception to this however, is doxycycline. The serum half-life of this drug has been shown to be unchanged in renal failure, and blood urea and creatinine levels have not been found to rise during its administration.

The administration of outdated degraded tetracycline has also been reported to cause a Fanconi-like syndrome.

8.4.3 Liver Toxicity

Excessive doses of tetracyclines can cause liver damage, and a number of deaths have been reported in pregnant women given large intravenous doses of tetracycline, usually for the treatment of pyelonephritis. See also section 19.2.4.

9. The Macrolides

Erythromycin, triacetyloleandomycin and spiramycin are the best known of the macrolide group of antibiotics so called because their chemical structure is based on a macrocyclic lactone ring. Originally produced by *Streptomyces erythreus waksman* found in soil in the Philippines, they were subsequently purified and first used clinically in the 1950's. The most widely used member, erythromycin, still enjoys an enviable reputation as an effective and virtually non-toxic antibacterial agent. A recent appraisal of erythromycin appears in the Scottish Medical Journal (1977).

Table V. Indications in which the macrolides can be considered one of the treatments of first choice

---

1. Otitis media and bronchopneumonia — where *H. influenzae* may be responsible *in addition* to streptococci, pneumococci and staphylococci
2. Secondary bacterial infection during respiratory virus illness
3. Pertussis — prophylaxis of, and treatment of bacterial bronchopneumonia
4. Alternative to benzylpenicillin or phenoxymethylpenicillin in hypersensitive patients who would otherwise have received a natural penicillin (see table II)
5. Staphylococcal infections of such severity that prolonged treatment is envisaged
6. Alternative to tetracyclines in *Mycoplasma pneumoniae* and T-strain infections

---

9.1 Erythromycin

9.1.1 Physicochemical Properties

Erythromycin is a whitish crystalline substance. With the exception of its gluceptate (glucoheptonate) and lactobionate salts, it is relatively insoluble in water but does dissolve well in organic solvents. Erythromycin salts are inactivated by acid solutions, except for erythromycin estolate (the lauryl sulphate ester) which is acid stable. An increasing pH therefore enhances the action of erythromycin.

9.1.2 Antibacterial Activity

The action of erythromycin depends on the sensitivity of the organisms and on the inoculum size. It is bactericidal in high concentrations and bacteriostatic at low concentrations. Erythromycin is thought to inhibit protein synthesis by interfering with ribosomal binding sites (Oleinick and Corcoran, 1969).

Spectrum of Activity
Streptococcus pneumoniae and *Str. pyogenes* are highly susceptible, but *Str. viridans* and *Str. faecalis* are rather less sensitive. *Staphylococcus aureus, Staph. albus, Corynebacterium diphtheriae* and the clostridia are usually sensitive, as are certain Gram-negative organisms including *Neisseriae* spp., *H. influenzae* and *B. pertussis. Mycoplasma pneumoniae* and T strains, but not *M. hominis*, are also sensitive.

Development of Resistance
Str. pneumoniae, Str. faecalis and *Staph. aureus* can develop marked resistance to erythromycin after sub-culturing, but this is moderately stable and the population consists of both sensitive and resistant strains. Resistance is rarely seen during suc-

cessful short term treatment but may occur when the drug is used over long periods of time to treat infections more difficult to eradicate, such as endocarditis. Cross resistance, which is probably plasmid borne, occurs with lincomycin, triacetyloleandomycin and spiramycin in strains made resistant in the laboratory, but erythromycin resistant staphylococci isolated from patients are not necessarily resistant to spiramycin and triacetyloleandomycin (Garrod et al., 1973). Strains showing this dissociated type of resistance, first described by Garrod (1957), are cells, the majority of which are sensitive to erythromycin but which become uniformly resistant not only to erythromycin but also to triacetyloleandomycin, spiramycin and lincomycin and group B depsipeptides when grown on a medium containing erythromycin. However, the organisms quickly become sensitive again after growth in the absence of erythromycin.

Lacey (1977) has recently reviewed the place of erythromycin in modern chemotherapy. The fear of resistance developing has been one of the factors responsible for the under use of this drug. The pattern of resistance seems to develop from a very few organisms which are resistant in a very few patients. When this drug is widely used in hospital practice these resistant organisms may multiply and spread but in general practice there appears to be no risk at all of this happening.

9.1.3 Pharmacology

Oral formulations containing erythromycin base must be enteric coated as the drug is inactivated by gastric acid. The stearate is acid resistant and is absorbed in the intestine as the base. The tasteless erythromycin estolate which also is resistant to acid, is absorbed as the ester and is then hydrolysed to pharmacologically active erythromycin base. Erythromycin gluceptate and lactobionate cause pain when given intramuscularly and are preferably given intravenously if an immediate effect is needed.

Peak serum levels of 1.1 to 2.9µg/ml occur 2 to 4 hours after a dose of 250mg erythromycin estolate orally (Bell, 1971) and a peak of 3.5 to 10.7µg/ml is obtained with intravenous injections of 250mg erythromycin gluceptate (Lake and Bell, 1969). With the exception of the estolate food usually reduces the absorption of orally administered erythromycin compounds. There is evidence that erythromycin estolate is more protein bound than the stearate (Wiegand and Chun, 1972).

Erythromycin diffuses throughout the body, but not into the CSF which is only penetrated when the meninges are inflamed. Bile concentrations are higher than in the serum but erythromycin estolate is less concentrated by the liver than the other salts. The drug penetrates into prostatic fluid and semen and has been shown to cross the placenta. Little erythromycin leaves the body by the kidneys and this makes the drug particularly safe in renal failure. Most of it is degraded in the body by demethylation.

9.1.4 Therapeutic Indications

Because of the similarity in antibacterial spectrum of penicillin G and erythromycin, the latter is used in the management of patients with streptococcal infections who are suspected of being hypersensitive to penicillin. Erythromycin has the added advantage of being active against some of the penicillinase producing staphylococci, and where these co-exist with β-haemolytic streptococci in the nasopharynx erythromycin is the drug of choice. Similarly, erythromycin may be used as an alternative to penicillin to treat pneumococcal pneumonia.

Erythromycin has also been successfully employed in the treatment of severe staphylococcal sepsis and was the drug of choice prior to the introduction of the isoxazolyl penicillins, lincomycin and fusidic acid. A disadvantage is that with long term treatment, resistance may become a problem (section 9.1.2). Rarely, if the estolate is used for more than 14 days, liver damage and cholestasis may occur *(vide infra)*. A combination of an erythromycin salt, other than the estolate, with another antistaphylococcal antibiotic may be safely used for staphylococcal bacteraemia and endocarditis.

In the management of middle ear infections where Gram-positive cocci or *H. influenzae* may be the pathogens, erythromycin is valuable. *Mycoplasma pneumoniae* organisms are more sensitive *in vitro* to erythromycin than to tetracycline and atypical pneumonia responds well to erythromycin treatment. Diphtheria carriers are better treated with erythromycin than with penicillin, although rifampicin may possibly be the most effective agent. In the prophylaxis of pertussis erythromycin is probably preferable to co-trimoxazole (see section 21.5.9) and is probably useful in reducing the contagiousness if given early in the course of the illness. Chronic prostatitis, staphylococcal and streptococcal skin sepsis, and severe pustular acne are also amongst the conditions for which erythromycin treatment should be considered.

9.1.5 Dosage

The usual adult dose of erythromycin base, stearate and estolate is 250mg 6-hourly by mouth. For erythromycin gluceptate, lactobionate and ethylsuccinate, the usual adult dose is 600mg to 2g daily in divided doses by intramuscular or intravenous injection.

9.1.6 Side Effects and Toxicity

Erythromycin base is one of the safest and least toxic antibiotics. Erythromycin propionate and estolate do cause gastrointestinal side effects in a few patients, but marrow, renal or neurotoxicity do not appear to have been reported. In renal failure only minor dose adjustments are needed. When erythromycin estolate and the closely related triacetyloleandomycin (see section 9.2) are given for longer than 14 days jaundice may occur with features clinically resembling viral hepatitis. Liver function tests suggest cholestasis but some hepatocellular damage also occurs, while an associated eosinophilia suggests an allergic element is present. The biochemical and clinical recovery is complete after stopping the drug but may recur if either erythromycin estolate or triacetyloleandomycin is administered again. Liver toxicity is not found with other salts of erythromycin or with spiramycin.

9.2 Spiramycin and Triacetyloleandomycin

The pharmacokinetic properties and antibacterial activity of spiramycin and triacetyloleandomycin are closely similar to those of erythromycin, but *in vitro* sensitivity testing suggests that they are rather less active than erythromycin (Kucers, 1972). As with erythromycin, gastrointestinal upsets are uncommon, except when large doses are given by mouth, and skin rashes are rare. Triacetyloleandomycin may cause jaundice in the same way as erythromycin estolate.

Spiramycin, alone or in combination with a sulphonamide, is currently an accepted form of treatment in toxoplasmosis. In all other respects however, these drugs do not offer any major advantage over erythromycin, although they can be considered as alternatives to it.

10. Lincomycin and Clindamycin

Lincomycin derives its name from Lincoln, Nebraska. The antibiotic was isolated from a soil organism *Streptomyces lincolnensis* found in this area and it was first introduced in 1963. Lincomycin differs chemically from most other available antibiotics. One of its derivatives, 7-chloro-7-deoxy-lincomycin, now known as clindamycin, is superior in antibacterial activity and is also better absorbed following oral administration.

10.1 Mode of Action

Lincomycin acts by inhibiting protein synthesis at ribosomal binding sites. This similarity in action to erythromycin may explain the closely related antibacterial pattern and also the cross resistance that may exist between the two drugs with certain strains of *Staph. aureus* (Sanders, 1970).

10.2 Antibacterial Activity

Gram-positive cocci especially staphylococci, pneumococci and most streptococci (except *Str. faecalis*) are generally sensitive to lincomycin but *Neisseriae* and *H. influenzae* are resistant. Thus its antibacterial spectrum, though similar to that of the macrolides, is not identical. Other organisms usually sensitive to lincomycin include *Mycoplasma hominis* and *M. pneumoniae* (but not T strains) and *Bacteroides* spp. Clindamycin has been shown to be much more active against staphylococci, pneumococci and *Bacteroides* spp. than lincomycin (Wagner et al., 1968; McGehee et al., 1968; Phillips et al., 1970).

Although lincomycin resistance can be induced relatively easily by passage *in vitro*, opinions differ about the frequency of resistance seen in staphylococci isolated from hospital patients (Garrod et al., 1973).

10.3 Pharmacology

Lincomycin is well absorbed after oral or intramuscular administration. Although food will delay and reduce the serum levels of lincomycin the absorption of clindamycin is not appreciably decreased by food, and serum levels are about twice those achieved after equal doses of lincomycin. Both lincomycin and clindamycin are widely distributed in the body and are found in cord blood and milk, although little gets into the normal CSF. They appear to be concentrated in bone and are therefore indicated in the management of acute staphylococcal osteomyelitis (Geddes et al., 1964, 1977). The MIC of sensitive organisms is quickly exceeded by the peak levels achieved in the serum after oral doses, and a 4 to 6 hourly dosage regimen is recommended.

Although only a small proportion of lincomycin (9% in 24 hours) is excreted by the kidneys, patients in renal failure may achieve very high serum concentrations of lincomycin. The excretion of lincomycin and clindamycin is mainly via the bile and faeces.

10.4 Therapeutic Indications

Although lincomycin and clindamycin are effective in the management of streptococcal and pneumococcal infections outside the meninges, the prime indications for the use of these drugs are severe *Bacteroides fragilis* infection, staphylococcal sepsis and, in particular, staphylococcal osteomyelitis. It would be unfortunate if their therapeutic efficacy became blunted by more widespread use for trivial infective disorders in the management of which significant resistance was allowed to emerge. It has been suggested that lincomycin and clindamycin should be combined with another anti-staphylococcal agent in the treatment of staphylococcal infections (Garrod et al., 1973), but in clinical practice this does not always seem necessary.

One of the attractions of these drugs in the management of osteomyelitis is that they may be given either parenterally or orally and for long periods of time without the development of serious toxicity — other than the possible risk of an acute colitis in a few patients.

10.5 Dosage

In adults the usual dosage of lincomycin is 500mg 6 to 8 hourly orally (avoiding meal times), or 300 to 600mg by intramuscular or intravenous infusion 8 to 12 hourly. The usual oral adult dosage of clindamycin is 150 to 300mg 6-hourly.

10.6 Side Effects and Toxicity

As clindamycin has greater activity against sensitive bacteria and is better absorbed (with or without meals) after an oral dose than lincomycin, it may well entirely replace lincomycin in the near future. In addition, it does not appear to be associated with greater toxicity. In severe renal failure the dose should be reduced because of the increased half-life of the drugs. In liver failure too careful monitoring of serum concentrations is important because of the high levels attained (see sections 20.1.7 and 20.2.4). If it is essential to use these antibiotics in these situations dose reduction is required, but if suitable alternatives are available they should be employed instead. With both drugs transient diarrhoea may develop in some patients and very occasionally an ulcerative colitis-like state can occur (Kaplan and Weinstein, 1968; Scott et al., 1973; Cohen et al., 1973). Here, despite normal barium enema findings, proctoscopy shows elevated cream coloured plaques superimposed on an erythematous mucosa that is either friable or oedematous. Pittman et al. (1974) regard the appearances of both lincomycin and clindamycin colitis to be indistinguishable from idiopathic ulcerative colitis. Colitis may occur after parenteral as well as oral administration. A final appraisal of both drugs must therefore be cautious. To avoid hypotension and vomiting large intravenous doses of lincomycin should not be infused rapidly (Novak et al., 1971). In all other respects, however, both lincomycin and clindamycin appear to be safe antibiotics.

11. Fusidic Acid (Sodium Fusidate)

This steroid antibiotic derived from *Fusidium coccineum* fungus is chemically related to cephalosporin P_1. The acid forms colourless crystals which are sparingly soluble in water compared with the sodium salt, sodium fusidate, which is highly water soluble.

11.1 Mode of Action

Unlike the cephalosporins and penicillinase resistant penicillins which inhibit bacterial cell wall synthesis, sodium fusidate inhibits bacterial protein synthesis (Harvey et al., 1966). This may explain the lack of cross resistance between sodium fusidate and the isoxazolyl penicillins and cephalosporins.

11.2 Antibacterial Activity

Staphylococci, including penicillinase producing and methicillin resistant strains, are mostly sensitive to sodium fusidate (Hoeprich et al., 1969). Other Gram-positive cocci including streptococci are much more resistant and with the exception of the *Neisseriae* and *Bacteroides* spp., Gram-negative bacteria are insensitive to sodium fusidate. Gram-positive organisms highly sensitive to the drug include *A. israelii, N. asteroides, C. diphtheriae* and *Clostridium* spp.

Although a few resistant mutants do occur amongst staphylococci and increase in numbers *in vitro*, this does not appear to be a major problem in clinical practice except in the treatment of burns (Lowbury et al., 1962). Nevertheless, it has been argued that penicillin should be given with sodium fusidate in the management of staphylococcal infections. In theory, the penicillin destroys the resistant mutants and sodium fusidate the remaining large population of sensitive organisms. However, this *in vitro* synergistic effect is not apparent in clinical practice and indeed antagonism of the two drugs is quite likely to occur (Garrod et al., 1973).

11.3 Pharmacology

Sodium fusidate reaches its peak serum level of 25 to 30µg/ml in 2 to 4 hours after an oral dose of 500mg (Godtfredsen et al., 1962). Some accumulation of the drug occurs with repeated administration of doses above 250mg.

Penetration is good except for the CSF. Therapeutic levels are found in most organs, including bone, and the drug crosses the placenta and can be detected in breast milk. It appears to be concentrated and excreted in the bile (Godtfredsen and Vangedal, 1966), but very little is found in the urine. Consequently no modification of dosage is required in the presence of renal failure.

11.4 Therapeutic Indications

Sodium fusidate is such a highly effective anti-staphylococcal agent that it should be reserved for the management of patients with severe staphylococcal infections.

There seems little indication in clinical practice to combine it with penicillin (O'Grady and Greenwood, 1973) or with methicillin (Jensen and Lassen, 1969), although both regimens have their advocates.

Topical sodium fusidate has been used successfully in skin infections.

11.5 Dosage

Results with different dosage regimens suggest that 500mg orally 8-hourly in adults, or 20 to 30mg/kg daily in divided doses in children, is sufficient. The diethanolamine salt for intravenous therapy is available in the United Kingdom and has been successfully employed when the dosage and method of administration recommended by the manufacturers has been used. In adults, the equivalent of 500mg sodium fusidate as the diethanolamine salt — dissolved in a phosphate/citrate buffer and added to 250 to 500ml normal saline — is given intravenously over a period of 2 to 4 hours and repeated 3 or 4 times in 24 hours (Murdoch, 1974). O'Garra (1968) gave intravenous fusidic acid to an 11-year-old and a 78-year-old in divided doses totalling 1 to 1.5g daily and Liddy (1973) gave intravenous fusidic acid to a small number of neonates. In neither of these reports was toxicity encountered.

11.6 Side Effects and Toxicity

Sodium fusidate is relatively non-toxic. Mild gastrointestinal disturbances and skin rashes have occurred. In normal clinical practice the steroid metabolic effects that might have been expected, have not been evident (Wynn, 1965). Toxicity from intravenous administration to neonates and older patients has not yet been recorded (O'Garra, 1968; Liddy, 1973).

In penicillin hypersensitive patients, sodium fusidate is a suitable alternative to the isoxazolyl penicillins in the management of severe staphylococcal infections.

12. The Urinary Antiseptics

12.1 Nitrofurantoin

A large number of derivatives of nitrofurfurane exhibit antibacterial properties, but few of these have been found commercially or therapeutically acceptable. Nitrofurazone is used as a cream or ointment for the topical treatment of skin, vaginal, ear or eye infections, and furazolidone has been used for the prophylaxis and treatment of gastrointestinal infections and 'travellers' diarrhoea'. The most widely used of these compounds is nitrofurantoin which is of value in the management of urinary tract infections.

12.1.1 Physicochemical Properties

Nitrofurantoin is a crystalline substance soluble in alcohol and water. Its solubility increases with pH but at the same time its antibacterial activity is reduced.

12.1.2 Antibacterial Activity

Nitrofurantoin is thought to act by inhibiting acetyl-coenzyme A, thereby interfering with bacterial carbohydrate synthesis. This mechanism may also possibly upset the carbohydrate metabolism of human nerves (Loughridge, 1962) [see section 12.1.6].

Nitrofurantoin is effective against many Gram-negative urinary tract pathogens such as *Esch. coli* and some strains of *Proteus* and *Klebsiella* species. *Pseudomonas* organisms however, are usually resistant. Gram-positive bacteria such as streptococci and staphylococci may be sensitive but the use of the drug is limited for these organisms as, with the exception of *Str. faecalis,* they are less likely to cause infection in the urinary tract and this is the only site where nitrofurantoin is concentrated sufficiently to be therapeutically effective.

12.1.3 Pharmacology

Orally or parenterally administered nitrofurantoin does not produce therapeutic serum concentrations in the absence of kidney impairment. The drug should therefore not be used in the treatment of systemic infections. It is thought that about two-thirds of an oral dose is metabolised by tissue enzymes, mainly in the liver, and the remainder is excreted in the urine. Urine levels can reach as high as 100 to 250μg/ml after standard oral doses, providing renal function is not impaired (Kucers, 1972). These concentrations are many times in excess of the MIC of sensitive urinary tract pathogens.

Toxic blood levels are reached in the presence of renal impairment and under these circumstances urine levels are too low for the drug to be effective for treating urinary infections. Premature or neonatal infants should not be given nitrofurantoin as they are liable to achieve toxic serum concentrations (Finegold and Ziment, 1968). After usual oral doses blood levels of nitrofurantoin in cord blood are generally less than in maternal blood, and consequently as maternal levels are low in healthy subjects there is little risk of fetal toxicity.

Tissue penetration in general is not good.

12.1.4 Therapeutic Indications

Nitrofurantoin should be considered in the management of urinary infection uncomplicated by the risk of bacteraemia, particularly in patients with recurrent episodes of urinary infection requiring long term prophylactic therapy. Care should be taken however, in any patient with a urinary infection who is likely to develop renal failure.

12.1.5 Dosage

In adults, doses of 100mg 6-hourly are sufficient for most sensitive urinary infections. Long term prophylactic treatment is given orally in doses of 50 to 100mg each evening; in many patients 50mg nightly is sufficient and this almost completely avoids side effects. Children should not receive more than 9mg/kg body weight daily (Finegold and Ziment, 1968), and infants below one month should not be treated with nitrofurantoin at all. Intravenous sodium nitrofurantoin has few indications and is not recommended, as blood concentrations after intermittent doses are no more therapeutically effective than when the drug is given by the oral route.

12.1.6 Side Effects and Toxicity

Minor gastrointestinal side-effects such as nausea, vomiting and less often, diarrhoea, are very common and militate against the usefulness of this drug.

Neurotoxicity
Peripheral neuritis is a serious toxic effect of nitrofurantoin and is most often encountered in those who develop high blood levels in the course of renal failure (see section 20.1.9). Even in the absence of renal impairment changes in nerve conduction have been shown to occur after 2 weeks of nitrofurantoin therapy in healthy volunteers (Toole et al., 1968). Any sign or symptom suggestive of peripheral neuropathy demands immediate withdrawal of the drug as recovery is not always complete.

Pulmonary Reactions
Acute pneumonitis and subacute pneumonitis with or without eosinophilia have been reported with nitrofurantoin. These conditions are usually reversible on stopping the drug but corticosteroid therapy may be necessary in some cases (Leading Article, 1969). However, chronic pulmonary reactions with interstitial lung disease may not always resolve completely, even if corticosteroids are given (Rosenow et al., 1968). The triad of impaired lung function, liver damage and autoimmune antibodies has been reported in association with long term nitrofurantoin therapy (Back et al., 1974).

Other Side Effects

The occurrence of cholestasis and hepatocellular damage can both cause jaundice in patients taking nitrofurantoin. Haemolytic anaemia, which is most common in patients with glucose-6-phosphate dehydrogenase deficiency, and megaloblastic anaemia have also been reported. Yellow discoloration of the teeth in infancy is thought to be due to repeated direct contact of the erupting teeth with the drug in the mouth.

12.2 Nalidixic Acid

Nalidixic acid, a derivative of 1,8-naphthyridine, is a synthetic chemotherapeutic agent unrelated to the other main antibacterial drug groups. Nalidixic acid crystals are soluble in dilute alkali. Burman (1977) has briefly reviewed some of the recent concepts regarding the antibacterial action of nalidixic acid. The exact site of action is still unknown. It is thought that nalidixic acid inhibits bacterial synthesis of DNA and may possibly interfere with the conversion of intermediate sized DNA fragments into high molecular weight DNA in the Enterobacteraciae.

12.2.1 Antibacterial Activity

Most Gram-negative organisms except *Ps. aeruginosa* and *Bacteroides* spp. are sensitive to 10μg/ml or less, but Gram-positive organisms are largely resistant (Garrod et al., 1973). Development of both *in vitro* and *in vivo* resistance has been demonstrated but after more than a decade of use nalidixic acid does not appear to be inactivated by specific R factors as has been the case with other antibacterial drugs (Burman, 1977).

12.2.2 Pharmacology

Nalidixic acid is well absorbed from the gastrointestinal tract and following an oral dose of 1g peak plasma levels of 25μg/ml occur in normal subjects — although there is much variation between individuals (Garrod et al., 1973). About 93% of the drug is protein bound (Zinsser, 1970), and *in vitro* studies suggest that it may interfere with anticoagulant therapy by freeing warfarin from albumin binding sites (Sellers and Koch-Weser, 1970).

Negligible amounts of nalidixic acid cross the blood brain barrier (Finegold and Ziment, 1968). It is excreted in the urine largely as a pharmacologically inert glucuronide, although sufficient of the active drug is present for it to be therapeutically effective in the management of urinary tract infections caused by sensitive organisms. Although there is little increase in the serum levels of the active compound in patients with impaired kidney function, glucuronide metabolites of nalidixic acid accumulate. Opinions vary as to the efficacy and safety of nalidixic acid in uraemic patients (Adam and Dawborn, 1971; Goff et al., 1968; Lowentritt and Schlegel, 1969; Stamey et al., 1969) but caution is advised. It should not be given to children under 4 weeks of age or to premature infants whose ability to metabolise the drug (glucuronidation) is poor.

Hepatic failure is also a contraindication to the use of nalidixic acid.

12.2.3 Therapeutic Indications and Dosage

Nalidixic acid has little place except for the management of sensitive infections of the urinary tract. In adults oral doses of 1g 6-hourly for 10 days are effective and long term prophylaxis of bacteriuria can be achieved with doses of 500mg or 1g given at night. Nalidixic acid has been used successfully by the intravenous route in Gram-negative septicaemia (Zinsser, 1970) but it has now been surpassed by other chemo-therapeutic agents in this situation.

Although caution should be exercised in the use of nalidixic acid in early pregnancy, Wren (1969) has reported no adverse effects to mothers or their fetuses treated with this drug.

12.2.4 Side Effects and Toxicity

Nalidixic acid is relatively non-toxic. There is a low incidence of gastrointestinal upset, rashes and phototoxic skin eruptions. Severe neurotoxic reactions such as grand mal epilepsy are rare and have usually occurred where high doses have been given to patients who already have a predisposition to seizures (Kucers, 1972). Less dramatic central nervous system upsets do occur but are reversible on stopping the drug.

Raised intracranial pressure with papilloedema and a bulging fontanelle has been reported in infants (Boreus and Sundstrom, 1967).

12.3 Oxolinic Acid

Oxolinic acid is a quinolone derivative chemically related to nalidixic acid and possessing a similar antibacterial spectrum. While cross resistance between the two drugs occurs, oxolinic acid is more active than nalidixic acid over a similar antibacterial range. Because of its longer serum half-life it is administered in a twice daily dosage regimen, but any clear advantage over nalidixic acid in clinical practice has yet to be established.

13. Cephalosporins

It is now over 30 years since Brotzu recovered the mould *Cephalosporium acrimonium* from Sardinian sewage. This produced a number of antibiotics, but from the clinical standpoint, cephalosporin C and its chemical analogues are so far the most important to have been developed. The important cephalosporins at present available for parenteral use are cephaloridine and cephalothin. For oral use, cephalexin, cephaloglycin and cephradine are now available; the latter can also be given by the parenteral route. The cephalosporins are active against a wide range of organisms and are almost entirely excreted by the kidney. They are active against staphylococci with intrinsic resistance to penicillin and against penicillinase producing strains and may be used alone in the treatment of infections caused by these organisms.

Apart from the differences in their route of administration there are also some differences in their degree of activity against the various Gram-positive and Gram-negative organisms, with the exception of *Mycobacterium tuberculosis* and *Pseudomonas aeruginosa* against which none is active. All cephalosporin derivatives act by inhibition of bacterial cell wall synthesis and are bactericidal. The drug level required to achieve a bactericidal effect in most cases is only 2 to 3 times that required for bacteriostasis. The basic structure, 7-aminocephalosporanic acid (fig. 5) is similar to the 6-aminopenicillanic acid nucleus.

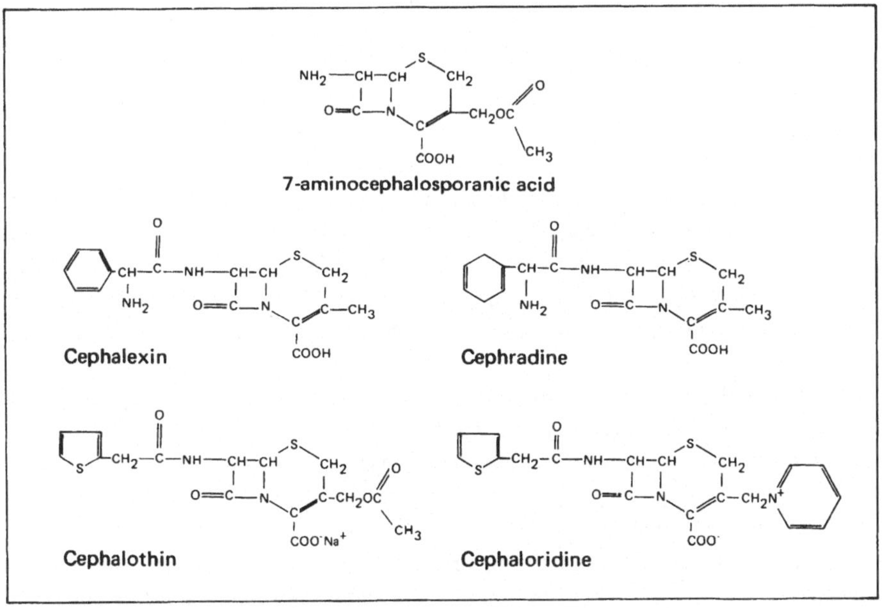

Fig. 5. Structural formulae of 7-aminocephalosporanic acid, cephalexin, cephradine, cephalothin and cephaloridine.

13.1 Cephaloridine

Cephaloridine has been in use clinically in the United Kingdom for almost 15 years and has been well documented (Murdoch, 1965; Eykyn, 1971; Leading Article, 1973).

13.1.1 Antibacterial Activity

Cephaloridine is actively bactericidal against a wide range of Gram-positive and Gram-negative bacteria but is ineffective against *Ps. aeruginosa*, enterobacter, indole-positive proteus and bacteroides. Its use is also limited against *H. influenzae* and *Strep. faecalis*.

13.1.2 Pharmacology

Since cephaloridine is not absorbed from the upper intestinal tract, parenteral administration is necessary. After intramuscular injection of 500mg, peak serum levels of more than 12µg/ml are reached within 30 minutes and adequate levels are maintained for up to 8 hours. Protein binding in the serum is slight (20%) and the drug is largely excreted unchanged by the kidneys, mainly by glomerular filtration. High concentrations in the urine are therefore achieved. The antibiotic penetrates well into inflamed muscle but very little appears in the bile or normal cerebrospinal fluid.

13.1.3 Indications

Gram-positive Infections
Cephaloridine is very active against *Str. pneumoniae*, *Staph. aureus*, *Str. viridans*, *Str. pyogenes* and *C. diphtheriae*. If the patient gives a clear cut history of allergy to the penicillins, cephaloridine should be considered as the primary treatment for *severe* infections caused by these organisms. Even in the patient with pneumococcal meningitis which is not responding to high doses of benzylpenicillin after 48 hours of treatment, a change to parenteral cephaloridine can be effective (Murdoch, 1965).

Cephaloridine by itself can be effective in the treatment of acute staphylococcal endocarditis but it cannot always be relied upon in this condition and combination with another antibiotic, such as gentamicin, may be necessary.

Gram-negative Infections
Because cephaloridine is active against *Esch. coli*, *N. gonorrhoeae*, *Clostridium septicum*, *S. typhi*, *S. paratyphi*, *S. typhimurium* and *Pr. mirabilis*, this does not mean that it is the antibiotic of first choice in infections caused by these organisms. It would not, for example, be indicated for salmonella infections of the gut. However, if the

patient is thought to have *Esch. coli* or *Pr. mirabilis* septicaemia, cephaloridine could be considered as the drug of first choice, especially in areas where there is no facility for monitoring blood levels of preferred choice antibiotics such as kanamycin or gentamicin.

Mixed Infections

These are especially liable to arise in debilitated hospital patients, particularly those receiving antimetabolites, corticosteroids or radiation therapy. Different organisms may be obtained from the blood on successive occasions (e.g. *Staph. aureus* followed by *Esch. coli* or *Proteus* strains). Here cephaloridine would be effective against all the likely pathogens with the exception of *Enterobacter* spp. and *Ps. aeruginosa*, in which case cephaloridine may be given in combination with gentamicin. There are objections to the use of this combination however, on the grounds of nephrotoxicity (see section 13.1.5) and in such cases it may be advisable to give cephalothin combined with gentamicin as this would be less likely to cause nephrotoxicity. On the other hand it should be remembered that serum levels achieved with cephaloridine are about 50 % higher than those reached with an equivalent dose of cephalothin (Eykyn, 1971).

13.1.4 Dosage

The standard intramuscular adult dose of cephaloridine is 500mg 6-hourly and this can be maintained for up to 14 days. For less severe infections, the dose can be reduced to 250mg 6-hourly. Intravenously, the dose is 250mg 6-hourly given by drip infusion.

13.1.5 Side Effects and Toxicity

In the doses recommended, cephaloridine is virtually non-toxic, but during the past 10 years reports of nephrotoxicity have been numerous. The nephrotoxic effect of cephaloridine on the proximal renal tubule is almost certainly dose related and is most likely to occur when very high serum levels in excess of $100\mu g/ml$ are reached. Usually, it has occurred with doses in excess of 6g daily in adults. Nephrotoxicity is enhanced by the concomitant administration of potent diuretics such as frusemide and ethacrynic acid (with which they should never be used) and by other potentially nephrotoxic drugs such as kanamycin and gentamicin. Patients with renal impairment are more prone to this adverse effect and the drug should be used with caution in such cases. An outpouring of casts in the urine is one of the first signs. It is probable that the nephrotoxicity is completely reversible by stopping the drug (Eykyn, 1971).

Excessive intrathecal doses, above 50mg daily, will cause drowsiness and mental changes, although administration by this route is seldom necessary in the absence of hydrocephalus. Intramuscular injection is virtually painless, but following injection, erythematous skin rashes can occur. This sensitisation is similar to the type produced by the penicillin nucleus but there is no convincing evidence that there is cross sensitisation between the penicillin nucleus and the cephalosporin nucleus (although this possibility should be remembered).

Cephaloridine remains a powerful, bactericidal, useful cephalosporin. It has been well tried over the years and, provided that excessive doses are avoided, the danger of nephrotoxicity is minimal. There is the added advantage over other bactericidal anti-Gram-negative antibiotics of non-toxicity in the absence of high serum levels caused by high dosage. If the clinician suspects a fulminating infection and the route of entry of the organism is certain, he can rely on cephaloridine as a powerful drug in this situation. This is particularly true when mixed infection is suspected and where the patient gives a clear cut history of penicillin allergy.

13.2 Cephalothin

Cephalothin is a semi-synthetic cephalosporin C derivative more recently introduced than cephaloridine. While it has a similar range of antibacterial activity to that of cephaloridine it may have some advantages over the latter. Experience with cephalothin is much less than with cephaloridine in the United Kingdom, but it has been much more extensively studied in the USA. There seems in fact to be little doubt that cephaloridine and cephalothin are highly effective antibiotics and have similar clinical indications. Cephalothin may be more effective and less toxic in higher dosage than cephaloridine, and this may have some advantage in treating very severe infections.

Like cephaloridine, cephalothin may produce skin rashes and may also be nephrotoxic in man, although to a lesser degree than cephaloridine (Eykyn, 1971). Excessive doses of either of these drugs by the parenteral route should be avoided where possible.

13.2.1 Dosage

Cephalothin may be given by either the intramuscular or intravenous route. An intravenous dose of 2.5 to 5g gives high blood levels which drop rapidly, and the dose interval should be 4 to 6 hourly for serious infections. High intramuscular doses of a similar range are also recommended for moderate to severe infections.

13.3 Cephalexin

Cephalexin was the first semi-synthetic cephalosporin C derivative which was shown to be absorbed from the upper intestinal tract following oral administration.

The range of activity of this cephalosporin is very similar to that of cephaloridine and cephalothin.

Cephalexin is not suitable for parenteral administration. Peak serum levels obtained after oral administration are variable, ranging from 2.7 to 19μg per ml after a 500mg dose (Eykyn, 1971). Cephalexin is only minimally bound to serum protein (about 13 to 19%). It is excreted largely in the urine and the administered dose can be almost totally recovered from the urine in 6 hours. As it is excreted mainly by the renal tubules, higher and more sustained blood levels can be achieved by the concomitant administration of probenecid.

The usual dose for an adult ranges from 250 to 500mg 6-hourly, but the dose may be raised to 1g 6-hourly in severe infections. However, it is not suggested that cephalexin is the best cephalosporin available. It is expensive and would not be used as primary treatment in place of ampicillin (or amoxycillin) or co-trimoxazole, for say susceptible urinary tract or respiratory tract infections. Cephalexin should not be given to patients with a known history of skin rashes following previous treatment with any other cephalosporin.

13.4 Cephradine

This cephalosporin is the first semi-synthetic derivative to be available in both oral and injectable forms. The oral preparation is very quickly and completely absorbed from the upper intestinal tract and binding to serum protein is only about 6%. Following intramuscular injection, peak serum levels of cephradine are reached within 0.5 to 2 hours (according to the dose), while the oral preparation gives peak levels within half an hour. Significant blood levels are present after 8 hours. The range of antibacterial activity is as for other cephalosporins (James and Walker, 1971).

Cephradine is suitable for the treatment of moderate infections caused by both Gram-positive and Gram-negative susceptible bacteria. For adults the usual dose is 500mg 6-hourly or 250mg 6-hourly for less severe infections. The paediatric dose is 25 to 50mg/kg daily in divided doses. Cephradine has been shown to be effective in both urinary tract infections (Butler, 1973; McLean, 1973) and respiratory tract infections (Mogagab, 1973).

The clinical pharmacology of cephradine has been determined and compared with that of other cephalosporins (Martin, 1973; Neiss, 1973).

13.5 The Cephamycins

As the cephalosporins are labile to the β-lactamases of many Gram-negative organisms, the development of the cephamycins may be an important therapeutic advance, since cephamycin C is less easily degraded by β-lactamases. Chemically modified semi-synthetic cephamycins are therefore being developed.

Table VI. Some properties of the newer cephalosporins and cephalomycins (adapted from Ball and Geddes, 1978)

Category	Compound	Route of administration	Side effects
Cephalothin-like cephalosporins	Cephacetrile	Parenteral	Eosinophilia, Neutropenia
	Cephanone	Parenteral	Eosinophilia
	Cephapirin	Parenteral	Positive Coombs test
	Cefazolin	Parenteral	Eosinophilia, Drug fever
	Cefatrizine	Parenteral and oral	Nil so far
β-Lactamase-resistant cephalosporins and cephamycins	Cefuroxime	Parenteral	Nil so far
	Cefamandole	Parenteral	Liver enzymes deranged
	Cefoxitin	Parenteral	Painful injection

13.5.1 Cefoxitin

Cefoxitin is analogous to cephalothin and its antimicrobial activity and pharma-cokinetic properties have been compared with those of cephalothin (Kosmidis et al., 1973). This showed cefoxitin to be more active against most Gram-negative strains, especially indole-producing *Proteus* spp., and in addition it was not susceptible to degradation by β-lactamase produced by Gram-negative organisms. However, it was considerably less active than cephalothin against Gram-positive organisms.

Blood and urine levels after injections of cefoxitin were also shown to be higher than after equal doses of cephalothin, and antibiotic activity in the serum was more sustained. No evidence of toxicity was found, and the authors concluded that the good pharmacokinetic properties of this drug, together with the lower MIC of most Gram-negative organisms and the lack of toxicity, are encouraging.

13.6 Newer Cephalosporin Derivatives

The new cephalosporins have been reviewed recently by Ball and Geddes (1978). This review has attempted to classify them using a clinical rather than a purely bac-teriologically approach; for details of these compounds the reader should refer to the original publication, but table VI summarises the main points made by these authors. In general terms it would appear that the cephalosporins tabulated have little real advantage over those previously described, with the exception of those showing stability to β-lactamases. Of these it might be worth mentioning the activity of cefuroxime against *H. influenzae* and *N. gonorrhoeae* and cefoxitin against indole-positive *Proteus* spp., *Esch. coli* and *Bacillus fragilis*. Nephrotoxicity has not so far been reported with these newer cephalosporins except in some animal experiments. It remains to be seen whether they will continue to be non-nephrotoxic.

14. Peptide Antibiotics (Polymyxin B and Polymyxin E)

Of the five polymyxins, A, B, C, D and E, originally isolated from a spore-bearing bacillus called variously *B. aerosporus* and *B. polymyxa* (Garrod et al., 1973), only two have found clinical usefulness, namely polymyxin B, usually in the form of the sulphate, and polymyxin E (colistin), either as the sulphate or sodium sulphomethate. They are basic polypeptides which are soluble in water and methanol and fairly heat stable.

14.1 Antibacterial Activity

The polymyxins act on the lipoprotein protoplast membrane by a type of detergent action causing increased permeability, swelling and rupture of the bacterium. Before the advent of carbenicillin and gentamicin, the polymyxins held pride of place in the management of *Ps. aeruginosa* infections. They are usually effective against *Klebsiella, Haemophilus, Aerobacter* and some *Escherichia* organisms, but are inactive against *Neisseria* and *Proteus* spp. Gram-positive bacteria are, in general, resistant.

There is complete cross sensitivity and cross resistance between the two polymyxins but not with other drugs. Polymyxin E is rather less potent than polymyxin B; most sensitive strains of Gram-negative organisms are inhibited by concentrations of 2.0µg/ml polymyxin B and *Ps. aeruginosa* is inhibited by concentrations of less than 8.0µg/ml (Smith, 1972). The development of resistance during treatment does not seem to be a problem.

14.2 Pharmacology

Polymyxins B and E are virtually not absorbed from the gastrointestinal tract. They are slowly absorbed after intramuscular injection, and therapeutic serum levels are achieved within 1 to 2 hours in the case of colistin sulphomethate and within several hours in the case of polymyxin B which appears to lose activity quickly in the serum. Colistin sulphomethate is converted by hydrolysis into colistin in the tissues.

Both drugs are excreted in the urine and toxic levels occur if the dose is not carefully monitored in the presence of renal failure.

Tissue penetration is good except for the CSF. In the presence of meningitis some polymyxin will cross the blood brain barrier (Smith, 1972) but combined intrathecal and intramuscular injections of the drug are recommended for *Ps. aeruginosa* meningitis if the polymyxins are to be used. Jawetz (1968) has stressed that colistin sulphomethate injection, which contains cinchocaine,[1] should never be used either intrathecally or intravenously, although polymyxin B sulphate and colistin sulphate can be used by this route.

14.3 Therapeutic Indications and Dosage

Polymyxins B and E work best when in close contact with susceptible Gram-negative bacteria in high concentrations — without any intervening tissue or membrane barrier. Topical administration for skin, eye, ear, joint, pleural or dural infections is ideal, and blood levels are sufficiently high after parenteral injection to cope with bacteraemia. Urinary tract infections also respond well as both drugs are excreted by the kidneys in therapeutically effective concentrations.

14.3.1 Topical Therapy

Topically applied solutions or ointments of 0.1% polymyxin B may be used to clear burned areas of pseudomonas organisms. Eye drops of similar strength or solutions for subconjunctival injection may be used when *Ps. aeruginosa* infects the eye after surgery. Polymyxin nebulisers containing 2 to 10mg/ml may also be successful in pseudomonas respiratory infections in patients with bronchiectasis or mucoviscidosis.

A 1mg/ml solution has been used to irrigate infected wounds. External otitis due to pseudomonas responds to 0.1% polymyxin B solution which may be combined with neomycin or bacitracin.

14.3.2 Parenteral Therapy

Parenteral polymyxin therapy may be needed in addition to topical applications of the drug and should always be used for urinary infections. Colistin sulphomethate is preferable to polymyxin B sulphate as an intramuscular injection as it is less painful and less toxic. Doses between 2.5 and 5.0mg/kg daily have been used. Colistin

---

1   Cinchocaine (dibucaine) is included in colistin sulphomethate injection in some countries and the formulation should be checked before it is given other than by intramuscular injection.

sulphomethate is not recommended for intravenous use but colistin sulphate, without added cinchocaine, or polymyxin B may be given by this route in doses of 2.5 to 5.0mg/kg daily by continuous infusion.

14.3.3 Intrathecal Therapy

In adults pseudomonas meningitis is usually secondary to trauma or surgery. Intrathecal polymyxin B in 0.5mg/ml concentrations may be given to adults in a single total daily dose of 5 to 10mg, or to children under 2 years, in a single total daily dose of 2mg. Colistin sulphomethate may be given intrathecally in a daily dose of 0.04mg/kg (500 units/kg) providing a preparation *without* cinchocaine is used.

14.3.4 Oral Therapy

Despite promising *in vitro* sensitivity patterns, oral polymyxins are not recommended for gastrointestinal infections due to *Shigella* spp. and salmonellae because they are disappointing in clinical practice (Marsden and Hyde, 1962).

14.4 Side Effects and Toxicity

Pain at the injection site is less frequent with sulphomethyl derivatives than with the sulphates.

14.4.1 Neurotoxicity

Neurotoxicity manifests itself in reversible paraesthesiae in the circum-oral and 'stocking and glove' distribution. Neurotoxic symptoms may even begin with blood levels of 1 to 2µg/ml (Jawetz, 1968). More serious is the apnoea associated with high blood levels of polymyxin which are reached in the presence of renal impairment. It is thought that the detergent effect of the polymyxins on bacterial lipoproteins may similarly work on the lipids in the synaptic connections of the nervous system (Naiman and Martin, 1967). Special caution should therefore be observed in uraemic patients or those receiving curare-like muscle relaxants or aminoglycoside antibiotics (see section 15) [Perkins, 1964; Prevoznik, 1967; Wolinsky and Hines, 1962]. The effects are usually reversible but assisted ventilation may be necessary.

Blood levels should be monitored and kept well below 10µg/ml. Levels of polymyxin B in excess of 5µg/ml make neurotoxicity very likely (Hoeprich, 1970).

14.4.2 Nephrotoxicity

Nephrotoxicity may also occur with the polymyxins but this can be avoided by not exceeding the recommended dosage in patients with normal renal function and by

adequately reducing the dosage in those with renal impairment or when other nephrotoxic drugs are being given concomitantly (Goodwin, 1970) [see also section
20.1.12].

15. The Aminoglycosides

Ten clinically important members of this group have now been isolated: streptomycin, neomycin, framycetin, paromomycin, kanamycin, gentamicin, tobramycin,
amikacin, sissomicin and netilmicin. All are chemically similar, as are a number of
experimental aminoglycosides not yet under clinical trial.

The aminoglycosides are poorly absorbed from the gastrointestinal tract, and
have toxic effects on the kidney and on the inner ear. Their spectra of activity are
broadly similar, with the exception of the activity exhibited against *Pseudomonas
aeruginosa* by gentamicin, tobramycin, amikacin, sissomicin and netilmicin, which is
not shared by earlier members of the group. *Streptococci* and obligate anaerobic bacteria are resistant to aminoglycosides.

In recent years transferable drug resistance has reduced the value of kanamycin,
gentamicin and tobramycin. This resistance is mediated by inactivating enzymes,
namely phosphotransferases, acetyltransferases and nucleotidyltransferases. The introduction of amikacin and netilmicin, which are resistant to degradation by some,
but not all, of these enzymes, has gone some way towards combating the problem.

The activity of the aminoglycosides fits them for use in serious systemic infections and, in the case of streptomycin, in the treatment of tuberculosis. Toxicity can
be avoided by careful dosage and correct monitoring of blood levels, especially in the
very young, the elderly and in patients with renal impairment.

15.1 Streptomycin

Streptomycin was first isolated in 1944 from *Streptomyces griseus*.
Dihydrostreptomycin, the product of catalytic reduction of streptomycin, is no longer
used because of the occurrence of severe ototoxicity resulting in deafness
(Christensen, 1960). The original wide spectrum of activity of streptomycin against
both Gram-positive and Gram-negative bacteria has now narrowed greatly due to the
emergence of resistance, and this has limited its usefulness. However, streptomycin is
still a 'first line' drug in the treatment of tuberculosis. Its use in this condition has
been reviewed by Crofton and Douglas (1969), and Ross and Horne (1976) [see also
sections 17 and 26].

Streptomycin has considerable toxic properties on the vestibular area of the
inner ear.

15.1.1 Antibacterial Activity

Streptomycin is active against *Mycobacterium tuberculosis*, many Gram-negative bacilli and some staphylococci. Resistance is common in the enterobacteriaceae and most streptococci are highly resistant (although enterococci are sensitive to the synergistic combination of penicillin and streptomycin). Partial to complete cross resistance exists between streptomycin, neomycin and kanamycin, but organisms resistant to streptomycin may retain sensitivity to other aminoglycosides.

Mode of Action

The mode of action of streptomycin, as with all the aminoglycosides, is essentially an interference with ribosomal peptide/protein synthesis at both m-RNA codon and ribosomal cycle stages. All the aminoglycosides are bactericidal. Garrod et al. (1973) consider that late effects on the cell, such as changes in permeability and respiration engendered by failing protein synthesis, may more fully explain this action.

15.1.2 Pharmacology

Simon (1968) has reviewed the pharmacology of streptomycin. The drug is not appreciably absorbed when given orally. After intramuscular administration doses of 1g produce peak blood levels in the region of $50\mu g/ml$. The serum half-life is 2.5 hours, and the drug is 30 to 40% protein bound. It penetrates poorly into the cerebrospinal fluid but appreciable quantities appear in bile. Transplacental spread occurs.

Streptomycin is excreted by glomerular filtration, about 60 to 90% of the dose being recovered in the urine. In older patients and in those with renal failure the drug may accumulate, and in the latter the serum half-life may be prolonged up to 50 to 100 hours (Kunin and Finland, 1959). Streptomycin is removable by dialysis and 'top-up' doses are required after dialysis. In premature or newborn infants the half-life is prolonged, varying with post-natal age (Nyhan, 1961).

15.1.3 Indications

Tuberculosis is now the main indication for streptomycin (see section 17).

Martin (1970) has extensively reviewed its use in other infections. It is the drug of first choice in plague and tularaemia when it is commonly combined with tetracycline (table VII). Its use in acute brucellosis has now been superseded by doxycycline or co-trimoxazole, and its use in combination with penicillin in enterococcal infections has been superseded by penicillin combined with other aminoglycosides (e.g. gentamicin). Streptomycin with chloramphenicol has been advocated as the treatment of choice for *Klebsiella pneumoniae* pneumonia. Simon (1968) suggests that streptomycin should be reserved for tuberculosis, tularaemia and plague.

Table VII. Indications for aminoglycoside therapy

Aminoglycoside	Treatment of first choice	Treatment of secondary or alternative choice
Streptomycin	Tuberculosis Plague Tularaemia *Klebsiella pneumoniae* pneumonia (in combination with chloramphenicol)	Brucellosis
Kanamycin	Serious Gram-negative sepsis: 　a) Septicaemia 　b) Pyelonephritis	Staphylococcal infection Tuberculosis (remains a reserve drug but safer effective alternatives are available)
Gentamicin	Serious Gram-negative sepsis, especially where the infecting organism is *Ps. aeruginosa* Enterococcal endocarditis (in combination with penicillin) Opportunistic infections in neutropenic patients (combined with clindamycin)	Staphylococcal infection requiring parenteral therapy
Tobramycin	*Pseudomonas* infections Other indications as for gentamicin	
Neomycin	Bowel sterilisation in hepatic encephalopathy (orally) Conjunctival and external ear infections (topical use only) *NB.* Neomycin, framycetin and paromomycin should *never* be used parenterally	
Framycetin	Conjunctival and external ear infections (topical use only)	...
Paromomycin	...	Intestinal helminthiasis Amoebiasis Possible use in shigella carrier states

15.1.4 Dosage

The intramuscular route is used. Young adults should receive 1g per day in single or two divided doses. Adults over 50 years receive a modified daily dose of 0.75g. In renal failure the dose is modified. Precise dosage schedules have not been formulated but Kunin (1967) suggests that the patient with anuria or creatinine clearance less than 10ml/minute should receive 0.5g at intervals of 3 to 4 days.

The dosage in children should be 20mg/kg daily and only exceptionally 40mg/kg daily. Intrathecal streptomycin in tuberculous meningitis in the majority opinion is unnecessary.

15.1.5 Side Effects and Toxicity

Severe vestibular upset is the hallmark of streptomycin toxicity, but deafness may sometimes occur. Vestibular upset manifests itself during the treatment course and is related to toxic peak serum levels and the duration of treatment. It is usually permanent. The elderly, neonates, patients with renal impairment and patients taking other ototoxic drugs are at high risk.

Nephrotoxicity
This is rare with streptomycin and is usually manifested by excess cellular excretion and mild proteinuria. Mild elevation of blood urea has been observed.

Neuromuscular Blockade
Instillation into body cavities, use during anaesthesia associated with neuromuscular blocking agents and overdosage in children, have all been associated with this complication. Martin (1970) considers it unlikely to occur in children if the dosage is less than 20mg/kg.

Other Reactions
Hypersensitivity (drug fever and rashes) are not uncommon and haemolytic anaemia has been reported. Intrathecal use has been associated with arachnoiditis. Optic neuritis may also occur (see section 17.1).

15.2 Kanamycin

Kanamycin is derived from *Streptomyces kanamyceticus*, and was first isolated in 1957. It is chemically similar to other aminoglycosides and is suitable for the treatment of severe Gram-negative sepsis. It also has important ototoxicity.

15.2.1 Antibacterial Activity

Gram-negative Bacteria

Kanamycin is widely active against the majority of *Esch. coli, Proteus* spp., *Klebsiella, Enterobacter,* the paracolon group, *Salmonella* and *Shigella* species. Dans et al. (1970) and Sabath (1969) have commented on increasing resistance in the group particularly in hospital infections. R factor mediated resistance is well recognised. *Pseudomonas aeruginosa* is resistant.

Gram-positive Bacteria

Although staphylococci are usually sensitive, Fujii (1969), Barber and Waterworth (1966) and Sabath (1969) have all described small numbers of highly resistant strains. Streptococci and most other Gram-positive bacteria are resistant.

Miscellaneous

Mycobacterium tuberculosis is usually sensitive, but resistance emerges rapidly (Dye, 1966).

Kanamycin resembles the other aminoglycosides in its mode of action causing ribosomal 'mis-reading' and disrupting protein synthesis. There is almost complete cross resistance between kanamycin, neomycin and paromomycin.

15.2.2 Pharmacology

Kanamycin is poorly absorbed from the gastrointestinal tract, and serum levels rarely exceed 0.5µg/ml after large oral doses. Intramuscular administration produces reliable serum levels maximal at 1 to 2 hours after a single injection, with a half life of 3 to 5 hours (Cutler and Orme, 1969; Kunin, 1966). No accumulation occurs in the absence of renal impairment. Peak levels after 0.25g intramuscularly may be expected to reach 12µg/ml (after 0.5g, 20µg/ml), falling to less than 4µg/ml at 6 hours. Children over 3 months have similar handling capacities, but the very young excrete aminoglycosides very slowly and accumulation may occur. Simon (1968) has reported peak serum levels of 17.5µg/ml in infants following injection of 7.5mg/kg, and calculated a half-life of approximately 9 hours (in neonates as long as 18 hours). Serum half-life was found to relate to postnatal age only.

Protein binding is minimal, and the drug is distributed in approximately 20% of body weight. Penetration into tissues is good except for bone and CSF. Little if any appears in the bile and stools (Kunin, 1966).

Kanamycin is excreted unchanged via the kidney by glomerular filtration, about two-thirds of the dose appearing in the urine within 24 hours. Urine levels greater than 100µg/ml can be expected for 6 to 8 hours after an intramuscular injection of 0.25g (Bunn, 1970). The renal clearance is 80% that of endogenous creatinine; up to 50% may be removed by a normal haemodialysis. Excretion is reduced in renal failure, the serum half-life having a linear relationship with the serum creatinine (Cutler and Orme, 1969). The half-life approximates to 3 times the serum creatinine concentration in hours, and dosage intervals of 3 half-lives can be calculated in renal failure. Cutler and Orme (1969) have shown that satisfactory blood levels are present if kanamycin is given in a dose of 7mg/kg every calculated third half-life (see also section 15.2.4).

Kunin et al. (1960) have shown potential toxic accumulation to occur after oral dosage in patients with both renal and hepatic failure and care must be taken in these conditions (see section 20).

15.2.3 Indications

Gram-negative Infections
Murdoch et al. (1966) and Petersdorf and Turck (1966) have confirmed the usefulness of kanamycin in serious Gram-negative infections, especially in the bacteraemias and pyelonephritis (table VII).

Staphylococcal Infections
Kanamycin resistance is becoming a problem and kanamycin has been superseded by lincomycin and the isoxazolyl penicillins.

Miscellaneous
Kanamycin is less effective in hepatic failure than neomycin and its use in bowel preparation pre-operatively has encouraged bacterial resistance to emerge in the very units where the drug has a major role in post-operative infections. All antibiotics are best avoided in gastroenteritis (see also section 15.5.3). Peritoneal instillation produces marginal benefit at the risk of neuromuscular block (see section 15.2.5).

Kanamycin remains a second to third choice drug for tuberculosis, but has largely been replaced by new oral agents.

15.2.4 Dosage

Opinions differ as to standard dosage intervals in adults. Murdoch et al. (1966) consider that 250mg 6-hourly for 10 days is sufficient to produce adequate blood levels and cure in most conditions. Cutler and Orme (1969) have suggested 7mg/kg at 12-hourly intervals and Bunn (1970) has approximated this to 500mg 12-hourly. Both regimens are effective, but 12-hourly dosage may carry a higher risk of acute toxicity following the higher blood levels produced by the greater individual dose.

Children should receive 15mg/kg daily in divided doses. In neonates and premature infants, Simon and Axline (1966) recommend a reduction to 10mg/kg daily divided into two 12-hourly doses in view of the prolonged half-life in this age group.

Dosages in renal failure must be modified in relation to the serum creatinine. In the Cutler and Orme (1969) regimen referred to above, dosages of 7mg/kg are given

Table VIII. Risk factors influencing aminoglycoside ototoxicity

---

1. *Endogenous*
   a) Neonates, young children, elderly patients
   b) Renal impairment
   c) Previous hearing loss

2. *Exogenous*
   a) Previous aminoglycoside exposure
   b) Exposure to other ototoxic drugs (e.g. ethacrynic acid; frusemide)
   c) Overdosage

---

every third calculated half-life; 3 half-lives approximate to 9 times the serum creatinine in hours. Healy et al. (1973) have suggested however, that this regimen allows prolonged periods of subinhibitory kanamycin levels and these workers have proposed a dosage schedule in which both the subsequent doses and the dosage interval are modified to obviate this 'trough' effect. Mawer et al. (1972) have constructed a dosage nomogram (based on computer analysis), for use in renal failure, requiring measurement of body weight, age and serum creatinine. Blood levels should not be allowed to exceed 32µg/ml (preferably 16µg/ml) and should be monitored one hour after administration. After dialysis a 'top-up' dosage of 7mg/kg has been advocated.

15.2.5 Side Effects and Toxicity

Ototoxicity

Kanamycin causes irreversible damage to the hair cells of the organ of Corti producing deafness (high frequency loss predominating). Kaneko et al. (1970) have also shown a contributory effect on Reissner's membrane. Ototoxicity is likely if peak levels of 30µg/ml are exceeded, but may also occur as a total dose phenomenon after a long period of administration.

Finegold (1966) has suggested that ototoxicity may be avoided if the dosage is not more than 15mg/kg daily (1g daily for an adult) and the total dosage period is kept short. Kass (1966) has reported a high incidence of chronic toxicity in patients treated for tuberculosis. Patients with renal impairment, pre-existing auditory loss or advancing age, and those receiving other ototoxic drugs are at special risk (table VIII). Serum levels and renal function should be monitored during treatment. Ototoxicity begins to occur after a total dose of 15g and is invariable after 50g (Bunn, 1970) [table IX]. It has been suggested that no patient should receive more than 40g of kanamycin in a lifetime.

Neurotoxicity

Neuromuscular blockade similar to that seen with other aminoglycosides has been reported and may lead to respiratory paralysis (Finegold, 1966). It rarely occurs with normal parenteral use but may follow intraperitoneal instillation (due to the high rate of absorption from this route). Other reported effects include headache, paraesthesia and an acute brain syndrome with hysteria and visual abnormalities.

Nephrotoxicity

Minor proteinuria, haematuria and excess cellular excretion occur. Occasionally a rising blood urea indicates major renal damage and kanamycin treatment *must* be stopped before prolongation of half-life exacerbates this toxicity. Kanamycin uraemia is reversible, usually over a period of months. Simon (1968) considers nephrotoxicity rare if the dosage is limited to 1g daily for 7 to 10 days.

Other Toxicity

Hypersensitivity reactions, usually with eosinophilia associated, have been observed. An intestinal malabsorption syndrome has been reported with oral administration.

Table IX. Aminoglycoside ototoxicity in relation to dosage

Aminoglycoside	Serum level which should not be exceeded	Total dosage associated with risk of ototoxicity
Kanamycin	30µg/ml[1]	15g (small risk) 50g (very high risk)[2]
Gentamicin	10µg/ml[3]	Not known, but likely to be quite small
Tobramycin	10µg/ml[3]	Not known, but likely to be quite small
Neomycin, Framycetin, Paromomycin	Should never be used parenterally[4]	

1   Serum levels of 30µg/ml are unlikely to be exceeded after standard 250mg 4 times daily dosage; may be more likely after 500mg twice daily dosage. *NB*. Care necessary in renal failure (see text).

2   No patient should receive more than 40g kanamycin in a lifetime.

3   Serum levels of 10µg/ml are unlikely to be exceeded after normal intramuscular dosage (3mg/kg daily in 3 divided doses) in patients with normal renal function (see text for dosage modification in renal failure). *NB*. Care in all patients if using intravenous route.

4   Absorption to toxic levels may occur in patients with renal impairment as a complicating factor in hepatic encephalopathy — serum levels should be assessed in this condition.

15.3 Gentamicin

Gentamicin was isolated in 1963 from *Micromonospora purpurea* and is similar to aminoglycosides isolated from *Streptomyces* species. It is a complex of three antibiotic substances and has important advantages over previously described aminohexoses, being exceptionally active against *Pseudomonas aeruginosa*.

15.3.1 Antibacterial Activity

Gram-negative Bacteria
Gentamicin is active against most of the Gram-negative species, including *Esch. coli*, *Proteus* spp., *Klebsiella* spp., the paracolon group, *Salmonella* and *Shigella* spp. (Waitz and Weinstein, 1969), but its outstanding feature is its activity against *Ps. aeruginosa* (Barber and Waterworth, 1966). However, resistance of this organism has been recognised since the early 1970's (Shulman et al., 1971; Snelling et al., 1971), and resistance rates of up to 20 % in the USA (Meyer et al., 1976a), and up to 5 % in the UK (Drasar et al., 1976) have been reported. Of equal importance in the USA is the emergence of resistance in up to 50 % of *Serratia marcescens* isolates (Meyer et al., 1976a), although this is not yet apparent in the UK (Gray et al., 1977).

Amongst other Gram-negative organisms from UK sources the overall resistance rate is about 1 % (Drasar et al., 1976). Resistance is due to transferable R-factors, originally reported in *Esch. coli* (Kabins et al., 1971), and *Klebsiella* spp. (Martin et al., 1971), and now widespread in bacterial species. These R-factors code for the production of aminoglycoside inactivating enzymes, 6 of which are capable of attacking gentamicin.

Gentamicin is inactive against anaerobic Gram-negative bacteria, and against *Ps. pseudomallei*.

Gram-positive Bacteria
Barber and Waterworth (1966) found staphylococci to be highly sensitive to gentamicin, including hospital strains resistant to neomycin and kanamycin, but resistance has now been reported. Streptococci are usually resistant but a combination of penicillin and gentamicin is synergistic against enterococci *(Str. faecalis)*.

Mode of Action
Gentamicin acts on ribosomal protein synthesis and has been shown in the laboratory to prevent incorporation of ^{14}C labelled phenylalanine into peptides, halting protein synthesis within minutes (Hahn and Sarre, 1969). The effect is reduced by high salt and calcium concentrations, and by pH changes.

15.3.2 Pharmacology

Gentamicin is not appreciably absorbed from the gastrointestinal tract, but systemic absorption may occur from the skin (McMillan, 1969).

Intramuscular administration produces a range of blood levels in individuals. Riff and Jackson (1971) have shown peak levels one hour after injection to be:

2μg/ml following doses of 1.5 to 2mg/kg daily
4μg/ml following doses of 3 to 4mg/kg daily
16μg/ml following doses of 5 to 8mg/kg daily.

Within normal variation peak levels may be toxic in 10% and subinhibitory in 30% of patients. Pennington et al. (1975), have shown that serum levels may be appreciably lower than predicted in febrile patients. Gentamicin is 30% protein bound, and is 10% bound to red cells. Later studies (Gordon et al., 1972) have challenged the figures for protein binding, suggesting that gentamicin is only minimally bound to serum proteins. Gentamicin is distributed in only 15% of body weight, mostly in extracellular fluid. Penetration occurs into bile, and pleural, pericardial and ascitic fluids, to about 30 to 50% of a simultaneous serum level, but cerebrospinal fluid penetration is minimal, except in neonates with meningitis (Riff and Jackson, 1971; McCracken et al., 1971).

Gentamicin is excreted unchanged by glomerular filtration in parallel with simultaneous creatinine clearance; Riff and Jackson (1971) have shown renal clearance of as much as 85% of the total daily dose. The serum half-life is approximately 3 to 4 hours. Excretion in young infants is prolonged and McCracken et al. (1971) have shown that in premature or newborn infants the half-life may be 3 times that in the adult. Suitable blood levels below toxic limits were seen after dosages of 1.5 to 2.5mg/kg daily and accumulation did not occur. However, these levels were subinhibitory for 20% of *Esch. coli* and the authors consider that 5mg/kg daily may be indicated in septicaemia.

The kinetics of gentamicin in renal impairment have been extensively studied. Gingell and Waterworth (1968) found that while peak levels were not influenced by renal function, the half-life in serum showed a linear relationship with the creatinine clearance. Similar findings have also been reported by Cutler et al. (1972) who have shown a more accurate relationship between half-life and serum creatinine. In normal patients, residual levels after 8 hours may be expected to be less than 1μg/ml but in renal failure accumulation will occur. Lockwood and Bower (1973) have observed prolongation of the half-life up to 53 hours in anephric patients.

Riff and Jackson (1971) have shown that gentamicin is dialysable at a rate of 60% of that of creatinine and Gingell and Waterworth (1968) suggest that for the patient on haemodialysis a twice weekly dose of 80mg after dialysis is sufficient.

Gentamicin has been used with carbenicillin as a synergistic combination against *Ps. aeruginosa*. However, McLaughlin and Reeves (1971) and Riff and Jackson

(1972) have drawn attention to a possible antagonism between the two drugs in that large doses of carbenicillin may inactivate gentamicin if given simultaneously. Noone and Pattison (1971) have reported inactivation of gentamicin mixed with carbenicillin in transfusion fluids, but not if the combination is given separately, i.e. if the gentamicin component is given by intravenous bolus injection. Riff and Jackson (1971) doubt that inactivation takes place in the patient and Winters et al. (1971) have shown that large doses of carbenicillin do not affect the blood level of gentamicin. However, in patients with renal failure, Ervin et al. (1976) have demonstrated a significant reduction in the elimination half-life of gentamicin when carbenicillin or ticarcillin were simultaneously administered.

15.3.3 Indications

Severe Gram-negative Infections

Gentamicin remains the agent of choice in these infections. Cox (1969) reported excellent results in infections due to the common urinary tract pathogens (except *Str. faecalis*), and Martin et al. (1969) found gentamicin the most effective therapy in Gram-negative septicaemia compared with cephalosporins, polymyxins and the other available aminoglycosides. Noone et al. (1974a,b) subsequently reported similar experience. Gentamicin is not replaced by later aminoglycosides, such as tobramycin and amikacin, as the clinical efficacy of these drugs against infections due to sensitive organisms is no better than gentamicin. Gentamicin is of proven value in infections due to *Ps. aeruginosa* and *Serratia marcescens*, but the emergence in some centres of significant levels of resistance amongst these organisms and others, may dictate the use of amikacin (15.6.2) where this is known to occur.

Staphylococcal Infections

Gentamicin is active against most neomycin and kanamycin resistant staphylococci (Barber and Waterworth, 1966), but resistance is appearing (Bint, 1976) and less toxic alternatives, for example fusidic acid and the isoxazolyl penicillins, are available.

Severe Burn Sepsis

McMillan (1969) has shown gentamicin superior to other agents in reducing mortality when applied topically to severe burns. Verdoglobinuria, associated with pseudomonas infection, constitutes an important indication. Resistance may occur after extensive topical use (Shulman et al., 1971) but usually regresses after withdrawal of gentamicin.

Enterococcal Endocarditis

The synergistic combination of gentamicin and penicillin or ampicillin has replaced penicillin and streptomycin in the management of enterococcal endocarditis, because of the emergence of resistance to the latter combination in recent years (Watanakunakorn, 1971). Experimental evidence also suggests that penicillin and gentamicin is more efficient in eradicating *Str. viridans* from infected heart valves than penicillin alone (Sande and Irvin, 1974). These factors, plus the activity of gentamicin against staphylococci, suggest that the most effective combination with which to commence treatment of presumptive bacterial endocarditis whilst awaiting bacteriological results will be benzylpenicillin and gentamicin (Schnurr et al., 1977).

Other Uses

Gentamicin has been used topically for ear and eye infections, but in view of the infrequency of *Ps. aeruginosa* as a causative organism, and the risks of inducing gentamicin resistance, an alternative agent, for example soframycin, is preferable. Oral gentamicin is of no value in gastroenteritis and should never be used. Recently, gentamicin combined with either lincomycin or metronidazole has been shown to be effective in the prophylaxis of postoperative wound infection (Feathers et al., 1977), but the risks of inducing gentamicin resistance are not inconsiderable, and these authors suggest that an alternative to gentamicin should be sought.

15.3.4 Dosage

Adults with normal renal function should receive 3mg/kg daily in three divided doses 8-hourly. In serious Gram-negative sepsis 5mg/kg daily may be needed to maintain inhibitory blood levels. The intramuscular route is indicated except when the drug is given in combination with carbenicillin *(vide supra)*. In renal failure, Gingell and Waterworth (1968) have proposed a scheme of dosage based on a range of creatinine clearances, but Cutler et al. (1972) consider that individual dosages should be calculated from the predicted half-life/creatinine relationship, and have shown the half-life to be equivalent to 3 times the serum creatinine in hours. Dosages are given every 2 to 3 calculated half-lives at 1mg/kg per dose. Barza et al. (1975), however, have questioned the accuracy of dosage prediction on the basis of the serum creatinine alone.

In neonates, McCracken et al. (1971) recommend a dosage of 1.5 to 2.5mg/kg daily but dosages of up to 5mg/kg daily may be needed in life-threatening infections. Older children may receive 3mg/kg daily (see also section 21.4.14). Newman and Holt (1971) have investigated intrathecal use and recommend 1mg per day intrathecally together with 2mg/kg daily intramuscularly in the treatment of Gram-negative meningitis.

15.3.5 Side Effects and Toxicity

Ototoxicity

The major ototoxic effects of gentamicin are on the vestibular apparatus. Wersall et al. (1969) have reviewed the evidence and shown progressive destruction of vestibular sensory cells. Cochlear hair cells are affected to a much lesser degree. Objective vestibular loss is always permanent but ataxia may be well compensated.

Ototoxicity is not only a peak level acute phenomenon (avoidable if blood levels do not exceed 10 to 12μg/ml) but also a chronic dose related occurrence. Jackson (1967) has suggested that the incidence of ototoxicity is approximately 2.5% of all patients treated with gentamicin. High risk patients include the elderly, those with renal impairment and those receiving other ototoxic drugs (table VIII). Jackson and Arcieri (1971), analysing ototoxicity, have suggested that in patients with normal renal function the total daily dose is the most important factor.

Nephrotoxicity

The total incidence of renal damage has been quoted by Falco et al. (1969) as being less than 2% of patients treated. Mild elevation of blood urea and creatinine, proteinuria and haematuria may occur, but are reversible. No relationship with either dose or duration of administration exists. Gentamicin should not be combined with cephaloridine or cephalothin, as the nephrotoxic effect of such combinations has produced renal failure.

Other Toxicity

Neuromuscular blockade may occur as with all aminoglycosides. Hypersensitivity is rare.

15.4 Tobramycin

Tobramycin is an aminoglycoside derived from *Streptomyces tenebrarius* and was first described in 1967. A complex of seven antibiotics — termed nebramycin — is produced by this mould of which tobramycin is the sixth component. Tobramycin has the advantage of being highly effective against *Ps. aeruginosa* and less toxic than gentamicin.

15.4.1 Antibacterial Activity

Gram-negative Bacteria

Dienstag and Neu (1972) have shown that tobramycin has excellent activity against *Ps. aeruginosa* and most enterobacteriaceae, and these workers have described strains of *Ps. aeruginosa* resistant to gentamicin that were sensitive to tobramycin. Various authors (Waitz et al., 1972; Waterworth, 1972; Britt et al., 1972) have reported up to 4-fold greater activity in comparison with gentamicin against *Ps. aeruginosa*, although Waterworth (1972) has commented on the greater activity of gentamicin against other species. Waterworth has also demonstrated synergy between tobramycin and carbenicillin *in vitro*, and has commented on the inhibiting effect of calcium and magnesium ions in test media on the *in vitro* activity of tobramycin.

Resistance to tobramycin is present in a significant proportion of isolates of *Pr. mirabilis, Serratia marcescens* and *Providencia* spp. *Pr. rettgerri* appears to be uniformly resistant (Britt et al., 1972). In 1972, Crowe and Sanders reported incomplete cross resistance between tobramycin and gentamicin, but it is now apparent that many of the R factor mediated aminoglycoside inactivating enzymes are equally capable of degrading both agents.

Gram-positive Bacteria

Del Bene and Farrar (1972) found uniform sensitivity of *Staph. aureus* and Britt et al. (1972) showed activity equalling that of gentamicin. Dienstag and Neu (1972) have reported that most strains of streptococci are resistant, but penicillin and tobramycin are synergistic against enterococci.

Mode of Action

Tobramycin acts on protein synthesis in a similar manner to other aminoglycosides.

15.4.2 Pharmacology

Oral absorption of tobramycin is minimal. After parenteral administration satisfactory blood levels are rapidly achieved and Black and Griffiths (1970) have indicated that peak serum concentrations, independent of dosage, might be expected 30 minutes after injection. Simon et al. (1973) have shown that peak concentrations of 2.4μg/ml and 3.7μg/ml are reached after dosages of 40mg and 80mg respectively and have calculated the serum half-life as 1.6 hours. Naber et al. (1973) however, have calculated a half-life of nearer 3 hours in patients with normal renal function, and shown that average peak levels of 6 to 7μg/ml are achieved after intravenous injections of 1mg/kg. Stratford et al. (1974), after slow bolus injections of 80mg and 1mg/kg, obtained average peak levels of 10μg/ml and 11μg/ml respectively.

Tobramycin has been reported to be 30 to 40% protein bound. Simon et al. (1973) have calculated a distribution volume of 15 to 17 litres, which is slightly higher than average extracellular fluid volume. The drug is cleared by glomerular filtration at a rate of 92% of the simultaneous glomerular filtration rate (Naber et al., 1973). Black and Griffiths (1970) found only 38% of the dose in the urine but Naber et al. (1973) reported up to 60% recovery within 6 hours. Urine concentrations vary between 20 and 80μg/ml (Simon et al., 1973).

In renal failure, Naber et al. (1973) have shown good correlation between tobramycin half-life and serum creatinine. As with gentamicin, Lockwood and Bower (1973) found a prolongation of the half-life up to 53 hours in anephric subjects. These workers have also shown that tobramycin is removable by haemodialysis to the extent of 70% reduction in serum concentration in 12 hours. 'Top-up' dosage is required thereafter.

In children, the pharmacology of tobramycin is similar to that in adults, except in the very young. Kaplan et al. (1973) showed that the serum half-life varied from 4.6 hours in infants over 2.5kg, to 8.7 hours or more in infants of 1.5kg or less. However, no accumulation was noted after dosages of 2mg/kg 12-hourly for up to 10 days.

15.4.3 Indications

Serious Gram-negative Infections
Tobramycin has established itself as a clinically effective addition to the aminoglycosides. Geddes et al. (1974) reported its successful use in a variety of invasive Gram-negative infections, including those due to *Ps. aeruginosa*, and Blair et al. (1975), found it to be as effective as gentamicin in *Ps. aeruginosa* infections. Tobramycin has been used successfully to eradicate *Ps. aeruginosa* from the sputum of children with cystic fibrosis (Hoff et al., 1974; Morrice McCrae et al., 1976). The worldwide experience of tobramycin has been summarised by Bendush and Weber (1976). It is primarily indicated in infections due to *Ps. aeruginosa*.

Staphylococcal Infections
Tobramycin is indicated in severe mixed Gram-positive and Gram-negative infections in which *Staph. aureus* is involved. Pure staphylococcal infections however, are probably best dealt with by lincomycin or an isoxazolyl penicillin.

Other Indications
Low concentrations of tobramycin encourage the appearance of resistant variants and topical usage, except in specialised units with problems of pseudomonas surface infection, should be discouraged.

15.4.4 Dosage

Naber et al. (1973) have suggested a dosage of 1mg/kg every 6 to 8 hours. Simon et al. (1973) recommended a dose of 80mg 8-hourly in adults. Synergy with carbenicillin against pseudomonas has been established, but inhibition *in vivo* may occur as with gentamicin (see section 15.3.2).

In renal failure, Naber et al. (1973) recommend that the dosage be modified to give standard 1mg/kg doses at intervals of 6 times the serum creatinine in hours (approximating to 2 to 3 times the half-life). Serum levels must be assessed frequently to prevent both under dosage and toxicity.

In children, 1mg/kg may be given 8-hourly, but in the neonate or premature baby 2mg/kg every 12 hours appears to be safe. Under dosage is as much to be avoided as over dosage as *in vitro* exposure of bacteria to subinhibiting concentrations results in rapid emergence of resistance (Waterworth, 1972).

15.4.5 Side Effects and Toxicity

Ototoxicity

Tobramycin is toxic to the vestibular hair cells of the inner ear at serum levels in excess of 10 to 12mg/litre. Continued exposure to high levels of the drug is probably more important in the production of vestibular toxicity than are isolated excessive peak concentrations, but Wilson and Ramsden (1977) have shown an acute reduction in cochlear output following peak serum levels in excess of 8 to 10mg/litre, indicating that auditory toxicity may be related to a peak level phenomenon. Ototoxicity due to tobramycin appears to be less than that attributable to other aminoglycosides (Brummett et al., 1972; Neu and Bendush, 1976).

Nephrotoxicity

Although tobramycin appears to be less toxic to the kidney of rats than gentamicin (Wick and Welles, 1967), the relative nephrotoxicities are less well assessed in man. Bendush and Weber (1976) found the overall rate of tobramycin renal damage to be 1.5%, which is comparable to the figures quoted for gentamicin (15.3.5). Abnormal cellular excretion, proteinuria, and occasional rises in urinary SGOT levels have been reported. Tobramycin should not be combined with other nephrotoxic agents such as cephaloridine or cephalothin.

15.5 Neomycin, Framycetin and Paromomycin

These aminohexoses are considerably more ototoxic and nephrotoxic than streptomycin or later group members and are not used parenterally. Neomycin was isolated from *Streptomyces fradiae* in 1949, framycetin (probably identical to neomycin B) from *Str. lavendulae* in 1953 and paromomycin from *Str. rimosus* in 1959. Their usefulness is limited.

15.5.1 Antibacterial Activity

All three drugs possess activity similar to streptomycin, and in addition paromomycin has helminthic and amoebicidal properties. Resistance to this group in *Esch. coli* and other enterobacteriaceae is increasing (Garrod et al., 1973), and there tends to be complete cross resistance with kanamycin. Staphylococci are now often resistant to neomycin (Leading Article, 1965) and streptococci are always resistant.

15.5.2 Pharmacology

Intestinal absorption is poor. Breen et al. (1972) reviewed the systemic absorption of neomycin after oral and rectal administration. Between 3 and 6% of the oral dose was found in the urine; no effect on absorption was found secondary to fasting, gastrointestinal ulceration or rectal administration. Similar absorption of paromomycin has been reported by Berk (1970).

Early studies of neomycin parenterally showed low protein binding and high renal clearance. Even after oral administration a very real risk of toxic accumulation exists in patients with renal failure (Last and Sherlock, 1960; Kunin and Finland, 1959). Berk (1970) has reported 5 cases of ototoxicity after oral dosage despite normal renal function. These antibiotics should be used with great care in neonates where the half-life is likely to be prolonged and toxic accumulation may occur.

15.5.3 Indications

Topical Treatment
Neomycin and framycetin are of proven value in eye and external ear infections and in some cases of skin sepsis, although sensitisation may occur. Staphylococcal resistance has lessened their usefulness in nasal carriage. The use of antibiotic sprays has encouraged the emergence of resistance with little or no benefit to the patient.

Gastrointestinal Infections
Neomycin has no place in the treatment of non-invasive salmonella infections (Association for the Study of Infectious Disease, 1970), and nor do other antibiotics. The carrier state may actually be encouraged by the use of antibiotics. Non-invasive shigella dysentery is not improved by antibiotics and Emond et al. (1969) consider antibiotics of little value in gastroenteritis of infancy caused by enteropathic *Esch. coli.*

Other gastrointestinal uses include:
1) Hepatic encephalopathy. Neomycin is the accepted agent for bowel flora suppression. However, reports of toxic absorption suggest that an alternative such as colistin might be used.
2) Pre-operative bowel sterilisation. Wound sepsis is only slightly influenced and the value of this measure is in doubt.
3) Lipid lowering effect. Oral neomycin may be of use in reducing hypercholesterolaemia (Today's Drugs, 1972), although it is not recommended that it be generally used (Levy and Rifkind, 1973).
4) Parasitic diseases. Paromomycin has a small place in the treatment of helminthiasis and amoebiasis. This drug differs from other aminoglycosides in being active against *Entamoeba histolytica.*

15.5.4 Side Effects and Toxicity

Ototoxicity

All three drugs cause irreversible deafness consequent on damage to the hair cells of the organ of Corti. Ototoxicity with neomycin may appear during therapy or progress after therapy is stopped (Leading Article, 1969), and may occur with oral or topical administration (Trimble, 1969). Kucers (1972) suggests that toxicity may be avoided if topical use is limited to the equivalent of 15mg/kg daily for at most 3 days.

Nephrotoxicity

Neomycin is very toxic to the kidney. Damage may be reversible.

Neurotoxicity

Neuromuscular blockade may occur as with other aminoglycosides, particularly after intraperitoneal instillation.

Gastrointestinal Side Effects

Apart from vomiting and diarrhoea, neomycin and paromomycin may cause malabsorption (Keusch et al., 1970) which may be due to an aminohexose effect on mucosal protein synthesis. Secondary staphylococcal enterocolitis has also been reported.

15.6 Newer Aminoglycosides

15.6.1 Sissomicin (Sisomicin)

Sissomicin is produced by *Micromonospora inyoensis* and is structurally related to gentamicin C_{1a}. It is active, but marginally less effective, against the same spectrum of organisms as gentamicin and tobramycin (Drasar et al., 1976) and is inactivated by a similar range of aminoglycoside inactivating enzymes. Blood levels and elimination half-life are similar to those of tobramycin; excretion, related to that of the serum creatinine — as with other aminoglycosides — is by glomerular filtration (Meyers et al., 1976b; Pechere et al., 1976). Toxicity in animals appears to parallel that of gentamicin, over which this compound does not appear to have any advantage.

15.6.2 Amikacin

Amikacin is related to kanamycin but is resistant to many of the aminoglycoside inactivating enzymes which have been identified, including those responsible for gentamicin resistance. Unlike kanamycin, amikacin is effective against *Ps. aeruginosa,* and is also active against many gentamicin resistant organisms (Reynolds et al., 1974), including *Serratia marcescens* (Meyer et al., 1975). Cabana and Taggart (1973) compared the pharmacokinetics of amikacin and kanamycin and found overall similarity. After a 500mg intramuscular dose, peak serum levels of 20mg/litre were obtained, and 80 % of the dose was recovered in the urine, the drug being excreted by glomerular filtration. The serum elimination half-life was found to be 2.1-2.4 hours. Howard and McCracken (1975) found the serum elimination half-life in infants to correlate inversely with postnatal age.

Amikacin has been used successfully in serious Gram-negative infection both in adults (Tally et al., 1975; Feld et al., 1977), and children (Howard et al., 1976) and appears a suitable alternative for gentamicin resistant infections. Toxicity is similar to that of other later aminoglycosides. For the present the use of amikacin should be restricted to gentamicin resistant infections, in which situations it is the drug of first choice.

15.6.3 Netilmicin

Unlike sissomicin and amikacin, netilmicin has not yet reached the stage of extensive clinical trial, however, advantages, *in vitro* and *in vivo,* suggest that it will almost certainly do so.

Netilmicin is closely related to gentamicin C_{1a}, and like sissomicin is derived from *Micromonospora inyoensis.* Its activity lies between that of sissomicin and amikacin, and it is resistant to some, but not all, of the aminoglycoside inactivating enzymes (Kabins et al., 1976). In animals, its pharmacokinetics are similar to those of gentamicin (Miller et al., 1976), but toxicity appears to be significantly less than with other later members of the aminoglycoside group (Luft et al., 1976). Should the findings in man prove similar, netilmicin may show itself to be the aminoglycoside of choice in the late 1970's.

16. Metronidazole

Metronidazole has been used effectively for many years in the management of protozoal infestation, both with *Trichomonas* and *Entamoeba histolytica.* However, although it was found to be effective in Vincent's angina some 15 years ago (Shinn, 1962), it was not until the recent upsurge of interest in anaerobic infection had occurred, that the agent became established as a powerful anti-anaerobic drug. Its activity, particularly against the obligate anaerobes, recently reviewed by Ingham et al. (1975a), places it amongst the drugs of first choice in these infections.

16.1 Antibacterial Activity

Metronidazole is exclusively active against anaerobic bacteria, strict aerobes and facultative anaerobes being resistant. *Bacteroides* spp. including the penicillin resistant *Bacteroides fragilis*, are highly sensitive (Nastro and Finegold, 1972) as are the majority of *Fusobacteria* and *Clostridia* spp. The effect of metronidazole is bactericidal. Anaerobic streptococci are also usually sensitive. Synergy has been demonstrated between metronidazole and both clindamycin and rifampicin against *Bacteroides fragilis* (Salem et al., 1975; Busch et al., 1976).

Amongst sensitive bacterial species, the development of resistance does not appear to be a problem. Ingham et al. (1975a) were unable to induce resistance in *Bacteroides fragilis* and considered the probable explanation of isolated reports of resistance to be taxonomic.

16.2 Mode of Action

Metronidazole acts as an electron acceptor in the oxidation of thiamine pyrophosphate by anaerobic bacteria, and the resultant compound exerts a bactericidal effect by interference with nucleic acid synthesis at DNA and RNA polymerase levels.

16.3 Pharmacology

The pharmacokinetics of metronidazole have been reviewed by Ingham et al. (1975a) and Hamilton-Miller (1975). Metronidazole is well absorbed from the small intestine and oral dosage of 200 to 400mg may be expected to produce peak serum levels of 5 to 10µg/ml within 2 hours. The serum elimination half-life is approximately 6 hours (Welling and Monro, 1972), 40% or more being metabolised to inactive derivatives, and 40% being excreted, unchanged, together with these metabolites, in the urine. The drug penetrates well into the CSF after large oral doses (Davies, 1967), and in variable concentration into breast milk (Gray et al., 1961). An alternative method of administration is by the rectal route, following which blood levels similar to those achieved after oral dosage are obtained (Study Group, 1975; Willis et al., 1976). An intravenous preparation is available from the manufacturers but is not released for general use. Intravenous administration results in sustained high serum levels, of the order of 20 to 30µg/ml, for at least 8 hours after a dose of 600mg (Selkon et al., 1975).

16.4 Therapeutic Indications

Metronidazole may be expected to be useful in those infections where *Bacteroides fragilis* and other anaerobes are the causative organisms.

16.4.1 Intra-abdominal Sepsis and Wound Infection

Willis et al. (1976) achieved a significant reduction of post-appendicectomy *Bacteroides* infections by the use of prophylactic metronidazole and successfully treated 5 postoperative anaerobic wound infections. The same study group (Willis et al., 1977), found a similar degree of efficacy, using metronidazole prophylaxis in patients undergoing elective colonic surgery, and successfully treated anaerobic wound infections which developed in 11 patients from their control group.

16.4.2 Gynaecological Surgery

The Study Group (1975) reported a marked decrease in anaerobic infection in a metronidazole treated group of women undergoing pelvic surgery and successfully treated 9 patients with non-clostridial anaerobic pelvic infection.

16.4.3 General Anaerobic Sepsis

Tally et al. (1975) have reported the successful treatment of anaerobic lung infection, and secondary cerebral abscess, with oral metronidazole, and Ingham et al. (1975b) have successfully treated anaerobic cerebral abscess *(Bacteroides* spp. and anaerobic streptococci), and septicaemia secondary to acute pyelonephritis *(Bacteroides fragilis)* and wound infection *(Bacteroides fragilis).* Recently Eykyn and Phillips (1976) have reported satisfactory results, in 50 patients with a variety of anaerobic sepsis, using an intravenous preparation.

16.4.4 Protozoal Infection

Metronidazole continues to be of value in amoebiasis, giardiasis and trichomonas infestations.

16.5 Dosage

In anaerobic infection oral or rectal dosage of 500mg every 8 hours should be used. Doses of 1g 6-hourly have been administered but doses of this magnitude appear unnecessary in practice. Eykyn and Phillips (1976) have given 100ml of an 0.5% isotonic aqueous solution (500mg) intravenously, over 20 minutes, every 8 hours with no untoward effects.

If pulmonary or cerebral abscess is the indication for treatment, benzylpenicillin, to which the non-*Bacteroides fragilis* anaerobic bacteria are usually more sensitive (Finegold et al., 1975), should be included in the regimen.

16.6 Toxicity and Interactions

Metronidazole has few side effects, of which mild gastrointestinal intolerance is the most common. Acute reversible neutropenia is described and a reversible sensory peripheral neuropathy has been reported following high dosage (Ingham et al., 1975a). Alcohol, taken concurrently, may precipitate a disulfiram-like reaction and should be avoided.

17. Antituberculosis Drugs

17.1 Isoniazid

This drug has been in use since 1952 and has outstanding, unique features in terms of low toxicity, easy absorption when given by mouth, followed by rapid diffusion throughout the body, and especially into the CSF. It also attacks tubercle bacilli in caseous or necrotic lesions and in cavities. It is very cheap. The standard adult dose for pulmonary tuberculosis is 200mg daily, which may be given as a single dose or twice daily. In miliary and meningeal tuberculosis, to achieve a high CSF concentration, the dose is increased to 12mg/kg/day. Effective blood levels are present for up to 24 hours after a single dose.

17.1.1 Toxicity

Toxicity with the standard dose is very rare but with the higher dosage sometimes required, peripheral neuropathy in the form of the burning hands and feet syndrome may occur. This can be combated by giving pyridoxine 10mg daily simultaneously. Other side effects are so rare as to be not worth detailing.

Isoniazid resistance will develop rapidly if the drug is given alone and the organisms will remain pathogenic for man, though perhaps with some reduced virulence. Nevertheless, there is no case for the use of isoniazid alone at any time. The drug is invariably used in combination (see section 26).

17.2 Rifampicin

Rifampicin is as effective a drug as isoniazid — possibly more so. Administered, fasting, in a single oral dose of 600mg it seemed at first to be devoid of side effects apart from tinting the sweat and urine orange. However, reports of jaundice occurring in patients receiving rifampicin have now been published. Its true incidence has yet to be assessed but in the meantime the drug should be used with caution in patients with a history of alcoholism or of conditions known to cause impaired hepatic function. Rifampicin is excreted in the bile in which the concentration may be 30 or more times that in the blood. Abnormalities of liver function tests, in the absence of jaundice, usually settle spontaneously and treatment need not be stopped. Enzyme induction in the liver interferes with anticoagulant treatment and also the efficacy of the contraceptive pill.

17.3 Ethambutol

Ethambutol is administered orally. Its important adverse effect is optic neuritis which is dose related. The recommended dosage is 25mg/kg for the first 6 weeks, and 15mg/kg thereafter. Sometimes 20mg/kg is used throughout. To facilitate flexibility of dosage the drug is marketed as 100mg and 400mg tablets. An expert opinion on the state of the retina should be sought prior to starting treatment. The patient should be instructed to report immediately if impairment of vision occurs, treatment being stopped at once pending assessment. Symptoms precede objective retinal changes. Recovery of vision is almost invariable. Rarely, drug fever, gastrointestinal upset or skin rashes may occur.

17.4 Streptomycin

The standard form used in modern treatment is the sulphate which can be given by the intramuscular route or by direct installation into body cavities. The oral route is worthless, as streptomycin is poorly absorbed from the gut. Section 15 should be referred to for further information about streptomycin and its use in other infections.

17.4.1 Pharmacology

Streptomycin diffuses readily into most body tissues but does not penetrate the CSF to any appreciable extent unless the meninges are actively inflamed. Excretion is by the kidneys and when renal impairment is present the dose should be scaled down to prevent high blood levels causing 8th nerve damage.

17.4.2 Dosage

The standard adult dose is 1g intramuscularly once daily. This may be reduced to 0.75g daily in combined chemotherapy and the dose may have to be modified still further, depending on renal function and whether the patient is over the age of 50.

17.4.3 Toxicity

As has been stated, especially in old persons, the 8th cranial nerve can be damaged by high blood levels, the vestibular component being more commonly affected than the auditory component. Damage to the 8th cranial nerve leading to dizziness can be compensated for in young patients, but in older people this is not easy, and in those over 50 years of age, and those with renal disease, the dose should be reduced to 0.75g daily. In patients over 60 years of age the serum level of streptomycin should not exceed 2µg/ml. The onset of tinnitus warrants the discontinuance of streptomycin at once.

Hypersensitivity reactions are not uncommon and these include skin rashes and drug fever, not only in the patient but in personnel handling streptomycin who can contaminate their skin by careless usage. The drug should be withdrawn on the appearance of any of the symptoms of skin disorder or drug fever. Eosinophilia and other blood dyscrasias such as haemolytic anaemia, hypoplastic anaemia and leucoerythroblastic reactions may also occur, but these are less common. Rare side effects include headache, flushing and vomiting after injection. Streptomycin introduced into the peritoneum or pleura may potentiate neuromuscular blockage produced by curare-like drugs during anaesthesia. Streptomycin may give false positive urine reactions with Clinitest but not with Clinistix.

17.5 Para-aminosalicylic Acid (PAS)

When given by mouth this drug is less active than streptomycin or isoniazid and its action is bacteriostatic. As the sodium or calcium salt given by mouth PAS diffuses well into body fluids and caseous tissues but does not reach the CSF. Within 5 hours serum levels are negligible. The original preparations of PAS were most unacceptable to patients because of the taste and gastric upsets, which were very common; the most commonly used preparation now is a cachet containing 1.25g or 1.5g of sodium aminosalicylate. Enteric-coated tablets are made for those who cannot tolerate cachets and granules are also available. Other preparations include calcium benzamidosalicylate, potassium para-aminosalicylate and phenyl-PAS. According to Ross and Horne (1976) however, modified PAS preparations should be looked on with some caution and judged against effective blood levels and the performance of the better established preparations. When PAS is given with isoniazid a daily dose of the sodium preparation of 10g is effective. PAS and isoniazid may be prepared in a single cachet or in granular form. The patient thus *has* to take both drugs, reducing the likelihood of resistance.

17.5.1 Toxicity

Gastrointestinal upset is common and can be minimised by taking the cachet with milk or an alkali towards the end of a meal. Hypersensitivity reactions are less common but include skin rashes, fever, disturbed liver function tests and, with prolonged treatment, goitre can occur with sub-thyroidism. In combined therapy with streptomycin, PAS and isoniazid, the drugs can be withdrawn and treatment with a corticosteroid preparation instituted; testing for individual drug hypersensitivity should detect which drug is responsible and the other 2 drugs may then be continued. If hypersensitivity occurs to 2 or 3 drugs, rapid desensitisation under cover of corticosteroids should be undertaken; it is rare for the patient not to be successfully desensitised thus. The skin rashes may be severe enough to cause exfoliation and intravenous hydrocortisone may be necessary to combat this.

Urine tests are available to detect whether the patient is taking isoniazid or PAS regularly. 'Phenistix' reagent strips will detect the presence of PAS in the urine; false positives may occur with aspirin or sulphonamides. The filter paper test for isoniazid in the urine detects only free isoniazid and may not be entirely accurate for individuals who acetylate the drug rapidly.

17.6 Capreomycin

Capreomycin is an antibiotic derived from *Streptomyces capreolus*, and is marketed as the sulphate. The normal adult dose is 1g given intramuscularly. Cross resistance with viomycin and kanamycin occurs, but not with streptomycin. Its adverse effects are similar to those of streptomycin — rash, giddiness and deafness — but in addition it has an important adverse effect upon the kidneys. Hypokalaemia, hypocalcaemia and hypomagnesaemia may occur, the patient complaining of profound lethargy and muscle weakness. Special care must be taken with this drug in the elderly and those with impaired renal function. Daily dosage should not be continued beyond 3 months, when the dose should be reduced to 2 or 3 times a week.

17.7 Other Drugs

Much less commonly used drugs are: thiacetazone given orally in doses of 2mg/kg per day; this may cause gastric irritation and blood dyscrasias: ethionamide and prothionamide given orally in doses of 0.75 to 1g daily may cause gastric upset and hepatic damage: pyrazinamide, 25mg/kg given orally, may cause liver damage, gastric upset and joint pains. These drugs are best reserved for difficult resistant cases unresponsive to modern primary treatment.

18. Chemotherapy of Gram-negative Bacillary Infections

18.1 General Considerations

The importance of Gram-negative bacillary infections is twofold. First these infections are often endogenous and so extremely common; secondly, if the infection results in bacteraemia, a serious or even fatal outcome is likely. Three American studies (Spittel et al., 1956; Finland et al., 1959; McCracken and Shinefield, 1966) testify to the increasing frequency over the past 4 decades of serious Gram-negative bacillary infections, both in adults and neonates, and to their persisting high mortality despite the advent of chemotherapy. Although there is some evidence of a return in the importance of Gram-positive organisms (Williams et al., 1976) infections with Gram-negative bacilli remain a serious problem.

There was no apparent change in the incidence or mortality from Gram-negative bacillary infections (Felty and Keefer, 1924; Herrell and Brown, 1941) in the years before sulphonamides or after their introduction. McCabe and Jackson (1962) stated that Gram-negative bacilli had become a major cause of hospital infection and in several large series mortality rates varied from 37 to 55% (Hall and Gold, 1955; Martin and McHenry, 1962; Maiztegui et al., 1965). When Gram-negative endotoxin shock complicates the septicaemia, fatality is high (Weil and Spink, 1958; Lancet Annotation, 1963). Weil et al. (1964) showed that endotoxin shock occurred in 169 of 692 patients with Gram-negative septicaemia. The mortality in this subgroup was 82%.

It is important to suspect the possibility of Gram-negative bacillaemia in any ill patient so that a prompt diagnosis can be made and the 'correct' antibacterial drug employed as early as possible. High risk groups include premature babies and neonates, the immunosuppressed patient — especially those receiving radiotherapy, corticosteroids or azathioprine — and those with diabetes mellitus, renal failure or malignant disease. Gram-negative bacteraemia is notoriously common during urogenital infection — especially after instrumentation — and in gall bladder disease and peritonitis. The patient's prognosis largely depends on the severity of the underlying pathology.

Blood, urine and any appropriate exudate must be promptly cultured and then the chemotherapeutic agent which will achieve bactericidal concentrations in the blood as well as at the primary site of the infection immediately prescribed. As the bacteriological diagnosis cannot wait the identification and determination of the sensitivity of the organism, treatment must be started at once, blindly, with the drug considered to be most appropriate. A prior knowledge of the probable sensitivity pattern of Gram-negative bacilli likely to be causing these infections, in any area at any time, is particularly valuable (Murdoch et al., 1966b).

18.2 Organisms

Excluding the Salmonellae, the Gram-negative bacilli most frequently causing bacteraemia are *Escherichia coli, Proteus* spp., *Klebsiella* spp., *Pseudomonas aeruginosa* and lastly, but with increasing frequency, *Serratia* spp. (Ball et al., 1977).

18.3 Choice of Antibacterial Agents

Until the advent of gentamicin, kanamycin was regarded as the antibiotic of choice (Murdoch et al., 1966b). Where *Klebsiella* and *Ps. aeruginosa* are considered unlikely pathogens, kanamycin still holds an important place in the therapy of serious Gram-negative bacillary infections. It has the advantage over gentamicin of a wider safety margin between the therapeutically effective and the potentially toxic doses. The spectrum of gentamicin, however, covers almost all the Gram-negative bacilli likely to cause bacteraemia and it is therefore widely used.

Gentamicin resistance is usually only found in hospitals (Sabath, 1969), particularly in burned patients (Shulman et al., 1971; Roe and Lowbury, 1972) and in those with malignant disease (Greene et al., 1973). Under these circumstances close monitoring of the resistance pattern, especially of *Ps. aeruginosa*, is essential. In time amikacin may be shown to be superior to other aminoglycosides when resistant species are suspected (Sharp et al., 1974).

In the seriously ill infected patient, combinations of antibacterial drugs may be justified until the pathogen is isolated and its sensitivity known. This is usually only necessary when it is initially not clear whether a Gram-negative or -positive infection is present or when there is the possibility of a mixed infection, as after severe trauma. An aminoglycoside combined with penicillin, lincomycin or metronidazole may be used. Where possible bactericidal drugs should be used in combination as synergism may occur. As antagonism can take place between a bactericidal and a bacteriostatic drug, if possible such combinations should be avoided.

18.4 Routes of Administration and Duration of Therapy

As a patient suspected of Gram-negative sepsis may suddenly become hypotensive and so not absorb drugs given intramuscularly, the intravenous route is preferable during the first 24 to 48 hours of treatment. Later intramuscular or even oral routes may be used for those drugs absorbed from these sites. A minimum of 10 to 14 days total treatment is recommended.

18.5 Precautions to be Observed During the Chemotherapy of Severe Gram-negative Bacillary Infections

Because of the risk of endotoxin shock with the sudden onset of hypotension, oliguria and even anuria, it is mandatory to observe the patient's blood pressure at frequent intervals and to chart the urine output. Dosage adjustments required because of the development of acute renal failure should be anticipated rather than awaiting the results of the serum concentrations of the antibiotic. When potentially toxic antibacterial agents are employed — such as the aminoglycosides, which are largely excreted by the kidneys — serum levels of the drug must be monitored regularly.

Disseminated intravascular coagulation is commonly associated with endotoxin shock. If anticoagulants are prescribed for its management, any alteration in the dose of the antibacterial agent may upset the anticoagulant effect with the risk of haemorrhage. Alternatively a rise in antibiotic concentration in the serum, secondary to the development of oliguria, may have a similar effect. Regular monitoring of the prothrombin time is therefore essential.

18.6 Specific Infections with Gram-negative Bacilli

18.6.1 Urinary Tract Infection

Esch. coli predominate as the most common infecting agent in all series, especially in general as distinct from hospital practice. *Proteus* spp. are next common with up to 13% of hospital infections being caused by these organisms (Murdoch et al., 1966a). If recurrent, *Proteus* spp. infections are often associated with renal calculus disease. *Klebsiella* spp., *Ps. aeruginosa*, *Str. faecalis* and *Staph. aureus* and *albus* are less frequently encountered. Mixed infections are rare.

Acute Pyelonephritis
Because of the frequency of bacteraemia, the management of acute pyelonephritis usually demands treatment with an aminoglycoside such as kanamycin or gentamicin, or one of the injectable cephalosporins. Treatment is begun as soon as blood and urine have been taken for culture. In uncomplicated first attacks of pyelonephritis, *Klebsiella* spp. and *Ps. aeruginosa* are unlikely pathogens and thus cephalothin, cephaloridine or kanamycin may be used. In a patient with known or suspected obstructive uropathy, or with a long history of antibacterial drug administration, gentamicin is more likely to be effective because of the probable development of resistant species. A 10 to 14 day treatment course is recommended with careful follow-up to exclude further urinary infection and a causative underlying anatomical obstruction.

Lower Urinary Tract Infections
The chemotherapy of lower urinary tract infections must be based on the isolation of the pathogen and the determination of its sensitivity. A drug which is excreted largely by the kidneys should be used. Soluble sulphonamides have been widely and successfully employed in general practice but are unlikely to be of value for hospital infections where 61% of the *Esch. coli* may be resistant (Murdoch et al., 1966a). In a large survey of pathogens causing urinary infection in general practice, McAllister (1974) found nearly 100% of the *Esch. coli*, *Proteus mirabilis* and *Klebsiella aero-*

genes were sensitive to co-trimoxazole and nalidixic acid; nitrofurantoin was almost as good. In a hospital unit dealing with patients suffering from recurrent *Esch. coli* infections there was little to choose between cycloserine, nitrofurantoin and sulphonamides, although fewer patients were able to tolerate the nitrofurantoin (Ormonde et al., 1969). Although cycloserine will not cover species other than coliforms, it is very effective both in short and long term treatment of *Esch. coli* infections (Murdoch et al., 1959; Gray et al., 1967). With attention to dosage at the extremes of life and in those with renal failure, very few side effects are encountered. Other drugs which have their advocates are ampicillin and cephalexin. Whichever drug is used, a 10 to 14 day course should be completed and urine cultures submitted afterwards to check for reinfection or relapse. A single urinary infection in a male patient, or more than 1 episode of urinary infection in a female patient, is an indication for radiological investigation to exclude obstructive uropathy.

18.6.2 Gastrointestinal Infections

The Gram-negative bacilli commonly associated with gastrointestinal infections are *Salmonellae, Shigellae* and, in infants, pathogenic *Esch. coli*. As a general principle it is now considered unwise to employ antibacterial agents for these infections unless the patient is severely ill or regarded as bacteraemic, as is the natural pattern in typhoid or paratyphoid fever. Under no circumstances should patients with diarrhoea of uncertain origin be given antibacterial drugs as this may exacerbate the condition and also lead to the development of multiple drug resistance.

Salmonella Infections

The chemotherapy of typhoid and paratyphoid fever should consist of a 14-day course of chloramphenicol in an initial adult dose of 4g daily reducing to 2g daily after the first few days. Sensitivity of *S. typhi* to chloramphenicol can no longer be guaranteed. Chloramphenicol resistance was a feature of the 1972 Mexican typhoid outbreak and multiple resistance is now encountered in some strains (Leading Article, 1972; Leading Article, 1973), although it is not yet a major problem in the United Kingdom. Where resistance is thought likely, either ampicillin 6g daily — partly intravenously or intramuscularly and partly orally — or co-trimoxazole (Geddes et al., 1971; Geddes and Goodall, 1972; Sardesai et al., 1973) should be used. Mecillinam intravenously followed by oral pivmecillinam is an exciting new alternative, especially when ampicillin resistance is likely (Geddes, 1977). [See also section 5.4]

The typhoid carrier is notoriously difficult to clear especially if gall bladder disease is present. Christie (1964) was successful, however, using large doses of ampicillin, fortified by probenecid, for 3 months. More recently, Jonsson (1977) has been successful in treating salmonella carriers with the new drug pivmecillinam (see section 5.5).

Non-invasive salmonella infections should not be treated with antibiotics as this tends to prolong the carrier state (Aserkoff and Bennett, 1969; Joint Project by Members of the Association for the Study of Infectious Diseases, 1970).

Shigella Infections

Gillies (1973) and Christie (1973) have reviewed this topic. As virulent organisms such as *Shigella dysenterae* are likely to show multiple resistance, sensitivity testing is important; however it is probable that the organisms will respond to gentamicin, kanamycin or ampicillin. There is rarely any need to prescribe antibacterial treatment for other forms of bacillary dysentery. Indeed organisms such as *Shigella sonnei* are often also resistant and there is the danger of inducing the further transfer of antibiotic resistance by the widespread use of antibacterial drugs for diarrhoea (Davies et al., 1970).

Infantile Gastroenteritis

Antibacterial drugs should not be given routinely to infants with gastroenteritis. Usually no pathogenic bacteria are found. Even when pathogenic *Esch. coli* are isolated there is little evidence that antibacterial drugs improve the acute condition of the patient or lead to a more rapid disappearance of the organism from the stools. Some workers do advocate chemotherapy in an attempt to reduce environmental contamination during a nursery outbreak of infection with pathogenic *Esch. coli*. The mainstay of treatment in infantile gastroenteritis remains the correction of fluid and electrolyte balance rather than the prescription of antibacterial drugs (see section 21).

18.6.3 Infections of the Biliary Tract

The most likely bacilli to cause biliary tract infection are *Esch. coli, Proteus* spp. and anaerobes. Apart from *Str. faecalis*, Gram-positive cocci are unlikely to be found as they do not thrive in bile. Although some antibiotics such as rifampicin, ampicillin and cephalexin are highly concentrated in bile, the amount of the drug present during biliary tract obstruction is so low as to have a negligible antibacterial effect. Without duodenal intubation or culture of T-tube effluent after bile duct surgery no accurate assessment of cure in biliary tract infection can be made.

As in all serious Gram-negative bacillary infections blood cultures must first be taken. The effect of either kanamycin or gentamicin on bacteraemia is usually so dramatic that rapid improvement of the patient's condition will follow despite the fact that these drugs are very poorly excreted by the liver. Investigation to exclude biliary tract obstruction must be undertaken as soon as the patient's condition permits.

18.6.4 Infections of the Respiratory Tract

Pneumonias

The most common pathogens in lobar pneumonia are *Streptococcus pneumoniae, Staphylococcus pyogenes* and *Mycobacterium tuberculosis*, but occasionally several different species of Gram-negative bacilli can cause acute life threatening pneumonias, particularly in debilitated or compromised hosts. Capsulated types of *Klebsiella pneumoniae* have a predilection for infecting the upper lobes of elderly alcoholic men. The patient is usually ill out of all proportion to the radiological or clinical evidence of his lobar consolidation. On the chest x-ray the horizontal fissure is bowed downwards and abscess formation occurs early. The sputum is often viscid and bloodstained but may not show klebsiellae. The mortality which may be as high as 50% is closely correlated with delay in starting appropriate chemotherapy. On clinical or radiological suspicion of a *Klebsiella* pneumonia, therefore, antibacterial treatment must be given before results of sputum and blood cultures are available. A combination of parenteral gentamicin and chloramphenicol is standard therapy for this condition.

Haemophilus influenzae alone seldom causes lobar pneumonia, but in hospitalised patients suffering from malignant disease, diabetes mellitus, cirrhosis or those receiving corticosteroids or radiotherapy, *H. influenzae*, coliforms, *Proteus* spp. and even *Ps. aeruginosa* may cause pneumonia. Penicillin with an aminoglycoside is often required for *H. influenzae* infections where sensitivity to ampicillin cannot be guaranteed. Gentamicin alone will usually be sufficient for coliform and proteus infections but again combinations of an aminoglycoside and a penicillin or a cephalosporin may be necessary. In pseudomonas infections high intravenous doses of carbenicillin can be used as an alternative to gentamicin.

Chronic Bronchitis

Acute exacerbations of chronic bronchitis are caused by pneumococci, *H. influenzae* and, less commonly, by other streptococci and staphylococci. The flora is often mixed. In hospital chemotherapy is traditionally given with parenteral penicillin and streptomycin, but if the patient is not severely ill oral ampicillin or tetracycline will be satisfactory, especially if the patient is at home and so less likely to have acquired resistant organisms. There is little firm evidence that continuous antibiotic prophylaxis throughout the winter reduces the frequency or severity of exacerbations except in those who have a very large number of infective episodes each winter (MRC Working Party, 1966; Johnston et al., 1969). Other workers (Malone et al., 1968) give the patient a supply of antibiotics to take for a week immediately he develops an upper respiratory tract infection or his sputum becomes purulent. This method is less costly and permits the rotation of antibiotics if desired. The cooperation of patients is mandatory.

18.6.5 Endocarditis

Infection of the heart valves by Gram-negative bacilli presupposes prior bacteraemia and the diagnosis rests on repeated blood cultures on appropriate media. In recent decades there has been a shift in the incidence of bacterial endocarditis which now affects the elderly more often than the young. Although *Streptococcus viridans* still causes most cases of infective endocarditis, other organisms include *Staphylococcus pyogenes* and *albus*, other streptococci such as *Streptococcus pyogenes*, *pneumoniae* and *faecalis*, Gram-negative bacilli and non-bacterial pathogens like candida and *Coxiella burneti*. Of the Gram-negative bacilli found in endocarditis, *Esch. coli* is the most common followed by *Klebsiella/Aerobacter* spp. and *Proteus* spp. (Weil et al., 1964). *P. aeruginosa* is uncommon. Other less commonly encountered Gram-negative bacilli are the brucellae and *Serratia marcescens*. The bactericidal effect of gentamicin should be exploited to the full in treating these rare but dangerous forms of endocarditis. As soon as blood cultures have been taken, treatment should be started with gentamicin 8-hourly with careful monitoring of the patient's blood pressure, urine output and serum antibiotic concentrations. The heart should be auscultated at least daily and the findings recorded, surgical advice being sought urgently if the heart sounds alter or cardiac failure supervenes. Treatment with an aminoglycoside should be continued for at least 14 days, after which a further 4 weeks treatment with less toxic drugs, such as the cephalosporins, ampicillin, carbenicillin, polymyxins or co-trimoxazole — depending on the sensitivity of the infecting organism — should be given.

18.6.6 Meningitis

With the exception of antecedent trauma, otitis media or sinusitis, Gram-negative bacilli, other than *H. influenzae,* are uncommon causes of bacterial meningitis in the adult. Treatment may be given with gentamicin, chloramphenicol or ampicillin. For neonatal meningitis see section 21.5.5.

19. Anaerobic Infections

Until recently the most widely encountered anaerobic infections have been those associated with clostridia. However, the growing importance of the non-clostridial anaerobic bacteria has been recognised over the past 10 to 15 years. In particular, infections caused by *Bacteroides* spp. and the anaerobic streptococci have assumed an importance that is having many therapeutic repercussions.

19.1 Clostridial Infections

Vaccination has lead to tetanus becoming a rare disease in many parts of the world. However, lack of compliance with vaccination schedules has increased the 'at risk' population. The development for use in passive prophylaxis of human anti-tetanus immunoglobulin with an extremely low risk of hypersensitivity reactions, has therefore been timely. Indications for its use are: those whose vaccination status is uncertain; those who have had an incomplete course of active toxoid prophylaxis, and those who had such prophylaxis more than 10 years previously. The treatment of tetanus consists of sedation and muscle relaxation using large doses of diazepam, and supportive therapy. Referral to a centre experienced in the management of the disease is mandatory.

Clostridial myonecrosis (gas gangrene) is an equally rare disease and other infections associated with gas production, including anaerobic cellulitis, anaerobic streptococcal myonecrosis and infected vascular gangrene, which may mimic it, are more commonly seen. Clostridial myonecrosis is characterised by an acute onset, severe pain and toxaemia, and relatively slight gas production. These features may be followed rapidly, especially in cases associated with septic abortion, by fulminating septicaemia accompanied by massive intravascular haemolysis. Treatment consists of excision of infected tissue, large doses of benzylpenicillin and the administration of polyvalent antitoxin. Hyperbaric oxygen therapy may be of value but mortality rates with and without this facility are comparable.

19.2 Non-clostridial Anaerobic Infection

Advances in laboratory isolation of anaerobes from clinical material have prompted a re-appraisal of the significance of these organisms in human disease. *Bacteroides* spp., fusobacteria, eubacteria, anaerobic streptococci and many other groups have been implicated in cerebral, pulmonary, intra-abdominal and pelvic abscesses, wound infections following general and gynaecological surgery, puerperal and postabortal sepsis, soft tissue infections, otitis media and otogenic meningitis, pyelonephritis, dental sepsis and endocarditis.

Non-clostridial anaerobes are part of the normal microflora of the mouth, bowel and female genital tract, and most anaerobic sepsis arises from these sites. Infections emanating from the mouth, for example pulmonary or cerebral abscess, commonly involve multiple anaerobic organisms, amongst which penicillin sensitive species such as *Bacteroides melaninogenicus*, fusobacteria and anaerobic streptococci tend to predominate. However, in infections originating below the diaphragm, penicillin resistant *Bacteroides fragilis* is the most common pathogen.

A variety of antibacterial drugs are effective against anaerobes, including metronidazole, clindamycin and lincomycin, erythromycin, chloramphenicol and co-trimoxazole. Benzylpenicillin is active against most of the anaerobes, but *Bacteroides fragilis* is resistant.

19.2.1 Pulmonary Infection

Aspiration pneumonia and lung abscess involve anaerobic bacteria in over 75% of cases, in half of which aerobic bacteria will also be involved. Although *Bacteroides fragilis* is a relatively infrequent offender in the respiratory tract, allowing the majority of cases to be treated with benzylpenicillin alone, the possibility of its presence should be considered in patients not responding to this therapy. In these patients, or in those in whom the presence of *Bacteroides fragilis* is confirmed, metronidazole 600mg 8-hourly by mouth, should be added to the standard regimen of benzylpenicillin 4 to 8 mega units/day. Aspiration pneumonia will usually resolve within 10 to 14 days of commencing the above treatment but lung abscess frequently requires 6 to 12 weeks treatment. Anaerobic empyema of the pleura may be treated similarly but the mainstay of treatment is repeated aspiration.

19.2.2 Cerebral Abscess

Anaerobic bacteria are the most frequently isolated pathogens from brain abscesses, *Bacteroides* spp. and anaerobic streptococci being the most common. Such organisms commonly emanate from the mouth and anaerobic brain abscess may complicate otitis media, mastoiditis, sinusitis, pulmonary infections, bacterial endocarditis, cyanotic congenital heart disease, trauma and surgery. Treatment requires prompt surgical drainage followed by antibacterial therapy. The possibility of infection due to *Bacteroides fragilis* renders treatment with benzylpenicillin alone hazardous and, prior to bacteriological confirmation, the patient should receive treatment to cover this possibility. Clindamycin does not penetrate the blood brain barrier and in the past chloramphenicol was commonly used. However, metronidazole penetrates the blood barrier in significant amounts and has been found to be effective in the management of cerebral abscess. Combination with benzylpenicillin or cloxacillin is required as metronidazole is ineffective against anaerobic bacteria, such as the frequently associated pneumococci, streptococci and staphylococci. Large doses of benzylpenicillin (2 to 4 mega units 6-hourly), and metronidazole (400 to 600mg 8-hourly), are required. If oral therapy is not feasible metronidazole may be administered by the rectal route. The period of treatment should not be less than 4 weeks.

19.2.3 Intra-abdominal Sepsis

The major role of non-clostridial anaerobes in the production of intra-abdominal, pelvic and wound sepsis is no longer in doubt. The infecting flora is commonly a mixture of anaerobic and aerobic bacteria, and chemotherapy must take this into account. It must also be emphasised that the primary management of many of these conditions is surgical and that without adequate drainage of the infection site chemotherapy is almost certain to fail.

Chemoprophylaxis of wound infection has been the subject of extensive debate, and the case for broad spectrum pre-operative antibiotic prophylaxis is, at best, unproven. Recently, however, metronidazole has been shown to be of value in patients undergoing hysterectomy and vaginal procedures, appendicectomy, and elective colonic surgery (see section 16.4). These patients were given 2g of metronidazole pre-operatively, and 200mg 8-hourly for 7 days thereafter. A significant reduction in postoperative sepsis was obtained as compared with control groups.

The isolation of bacteria from a wound does not necessarily indicate a need for antibacterial chemotherapy. In many cases the presence of bacteria within a wound represents colonisation following contamination at operation, and in others, even when pus is present, the infection may be at a superficial level without tissue invasion. Neither of these situations demands antibacterial therapy. However, signs of invasive infection of the wound margins, systemic upset or possible secondary septicaemia are indications for chemotherapy, but this does not replace the need for adequate drainage. Swabs and blood for both anaerobic and aerobic culture, should always be obtained before beginning treatment. A combination of gentamicin, 5mg/kg/day in 3 divided 8-hourly doses (dependent on renal function: see section 15.3.4), and metronidazole 400 to 600mg, or clindamycin 300 to 600mg, 8-hourly, will normally provide satisfactory cover until precise sensitivities are available.

The treatment of peritonitis and intra-abdominal abscess is essentially surgical, but the high incidence of attendant septicaemia provides a rationale for the use of antibacterial therapy in a proportion of cases. The routine use of broad spectrum therapy after minor peritoneal soiling at operation, however, is more likely to compound problems than to solve them. Serious sepsis is frequently caused by a mixed flora, in which anaerobic bacteria tend to predominate. Early systemic invasion is due to aerobes such as *Esch. coli, Proteus* and *Klebsiella* spp., but later manifestations, including abscess formation, are more often due to mixed anaerobic bacteria, such as *Bacteroides fragilis*, anaerobic streptococci and *Clostridium* spp. However, until bacteriological results are available, a regimen such as that suggested for invasive wound infection may be used, and modified thereafter with the assistance of the bacteriologist. It should be remembered that this form of therapy may mask deep-seated sepsis such as liver or subphrenic abscess, allowing recrudescence of pyrexia and systemic upset following its withdrawal. Failure of antibacterial chemotherapy in this circumstance indicates the need for further surgical intervention and not for alternative antibacterials.

19.2.4 Female Genital Tract Infection

Anaerobic bacteria are isolated from infections in this site in over two thirds of all cases. *Bacteroides* spp. and anaerobic streptococci predominate. The role of clostridia in postabortal sepsis has been referred to (see section 19.1).

Endometritis, acute salpingitis and tubo-ovarian abscess, bartholinitis and infections following vaginal and uterine surgery, are all likely to be due to anaerobes emanating from their commensal site in the vagina. Penicillin resistant species predominate in all but acute salpingitis, in which aerobes including streptococci, coliforms and gonococci are more common. Thus with this exception, treatment with clindamycin or metronidazole will be more likely to be effective than the commonly used ampicillin or tetracyclines. However, in view of the possible presence of metronidazole resistant aerobic cocci, clindamycin is the drug of choice. Clindamycin has serious side effects and should never be used for trivial indications (see section 10.6).

19.2.5 Other Anaerobic Infections

Infections in and around the mouth are frequently due to invasion by anaerobic oral commensals. Vincent's angina is a classical example and responds rapidly to a small (200mg 8-hourly) dose of metronidazole. Ludwig's angina, which may be due to anaerobic streptococci, responds somewhat less rapidly to benzylpenicillin. Synergistic anaerobic stomatitis, associated with diminished host defences, may be dramatically influenced by metronidazole in full dosage (400 to 600mg 8-hourly). Dental abscesses have been satisfactorily treated with metronidazole.

Anaerobes are relatively infrequently the cause of bacterial endocarditis, however when they are, penicillin sensitive species are most commonly isolated, allowing bactericidal therapy to be used. Metronidazole which, unlike clindamycin, is also bactericidal, may prove to be of value in penicillin resistant disease.

Non-clostridial anaerobic soft tissue infection includes mild local invasion around skin ulcers, anaerobic cellulitis, infected vascular gangrene and synergistic bacterial gangrene. As with clostridial myonecrosis, many of these infections require excision of infected tissue. Antibacterial therapy should cover the anaerobic bacteria and skin commensals such as staphylococci and streptococci which are frequently involved. Clindamycin is the agent of choice whilst bacteriological advice is awaited.

20. Antibacterial Therapy in Renal and Hepatic Disease

Special precautions are needed in the chemotherapy of the premature and newborn infant whose renal and hepatic function is not fully developed. This subject is dealt with separately (see section 21). Because of the increased likelihood of infection occurring in patients with renal and hepatic insufficiency, and because of the serious nature of infection in these compromised patients, an understanding of the use of antibacterial drugs in these situations is very important if toxic effects are to be avoided.

20.1 Renal Disease

The subject of antibacterial agents in renal failure has been admirably summarised by Garrod et al. (1973) who make a variety of important observations which serve as principles of therapy in this difficult area. First, the likelihood of toxic accumulation is higher in antimicrobials, such as aminoglycosides, which rely almost entirely upon renal excretion than for drugs, such as fusidic acid, which are largely eliminated by other routes. With some antibacterial agents, for example, nalidixic acid, there is a risk of accumulation in renal failure, not of the active drug itself, but of potentially toxic metabolic products. Nephrotoxic agents must be used with extreme caution in renal decompensation and especially when a urinary infection is being treated. Finally, the patient with septicaemia, in whom renal failure may be precipitated suddenly and dramatically, requires very frequent monitoring of serum concentrations of antibacterial agents if serious toxicity is to be avoided.

Drugs such as erythromycin, novobiocin and fusidic acid require no adjustment of dose in renal failure. Agents such as the penicillins, which are largely excreted in the urine in health, do accumulate but only usually require minor dose adjustments because their degree of toxicity is low, even at high concentrations. The aminoglycosides, polypeptide antibiotics, vancomycin, PAS and amphotericin B must be given in smaller than normal doses in renal failure to avoid toxicity. Yet other drugs including the tetracyclines (except docycycline), nitrofurantoin, cephaloridine (especially with concomitant frusemide) and chloramphenicol, are best avoided in renal failure if suitable alternatives are available.

Kunin (1967) suggests that the best approach to the patient with renal disease who needs an antibiotic is first to assess renal function. Those with a creatinine clearance of less than 10ml/min should be classed along with those who are anuric. The best agent or combination of agents should be selected for the infection without allowing potential toxicity to interfere with the choice. Then the full loading dose is injected with one half the loading dose given at stated time intervals as follows: 8 to 10 hours for the penicillins, 12 hours for lincomycin, 24 hours for cephalothin and cephaloridine, 3 to 4 days for the tetracyclines, kanamycin, streptomycin, polymyxin B and colistin and 9 days for vancomycin. The delivery of doses of antibacterial drugs at ever increasing time gaps however has disadvantages and O'Grady (1971) points out that the serum concentration may fall below what is therapeutically adequate.

20.1.1 Sulphonamides

Fischer (1972) found sulphadimidine was protein bound to a lesser degree in uraemic subjects than in normal controls. The mean excretion rate of sulphadimidine after a single intravenous dose of 1g was significantly lower in the uraemic patients who had considerable plasma levels of sulphadimidine remaining at 24 hours whereas the plasma level of sulphadimidine in controls was undetectable at this time.

It was concluded that a serious risk of drug accumulation existed in renal failure. Short courses of sulphonamides are probably justified in uraemic subjects, if considered essential, but blood levels must be checked.

20.1.2 Penicillins

As very high levels of penicillin G are achieved in uraemic patients (Plaut et al., 1969) and can be toxic, some reduction in dosage is desirable in renal failure. Methicillin, cloxacillin, dicloxacillin and flucloxacillin can be given safely in doses of 1 to 2g 8- to 12-hourly but oxacillin may be given more frequently in doses of 1g 4- to 6-hourly because its half-life is significantly shorter than that of methicillin and the other isoxazolyl penicillins (Bulger et al., 1964). Ampicillin rashes may be more frequent in patients with renal failure. Carbenicillin may be given in intravenous doses of 2g 8-hourly to patients with a creatinine clearance of less than 5ml/min. In the haemodialysed patient a dose of carbenicillin of 2g 4-hourly or, in the peritoneally dialysed, a dose of 2g 6-hourly intravenously is suggested by Eastwood and Curtis (1968). Penicillin, ampicillin and cloxacillin, however, are not significantly removed during haemodialysis.

20.1.3 Co-trimoxazole

Trimethoprim and creatinine are cleared at approximately the same rates but the serum half-life of trimethoprim is doubled when the half-life of sulphamethoxazole is tripled in renal failure. Welling et al. (1973) suggest that the combination may be given in renal failure in 12-hourly doses with the amount of trimethoprim reduced to one half and that of sulphamethoxazole to one third of normal. Because of this difficulty of dose adjustment and the fact that other agents are equally effective, co-trimoxazole should probably not be used in severely uraemic patients.

20.1.4 Chloramphenicol

Although active chloramphenicol does not accumulate in the uraemic patient, its metabolites do and the possibility of them causing bone marrow toxicity cannot be ignored. However, if doses are reduced, the therapeutic effect is largely lost. Kunin (1967) recommends that the normal dose be given in renal failure but many authorities feel chloramphenicol should be avoided altogether in uraemic patients. Haemodialysis only removes a little of the active drug so that dose modifications are unnecessary for the patient undergoing artificial kidney treatment.

20.1.5 Tetracyclines

With the exception of doxycycline, the half-life of which is not prolonged in renal decompensation, tetracyclines are contraindicated in uraemia for they may precipitate terminal renal failure (Leading Article, 1972). Clinical and biochemical deterioration is largely caused by the antianabolic effect which interferes with protein synthesis and increases the amino acid load for the failing kidneys to excrete. Some direct renal toxicity may also occur especially during pregnancy and in those with concomitant liver failure (Lew and French, 1966).

20.1.6 Macrolides

Although the serum half-life of erythromycin is a little prolonged in renal failure, only minor adjustments of dosage are required even in anuric patients (Kunin, 1967).

20.1.7 Lincomycin and Clindamycin

If renal failure is severe the dose should be reduced because the serum half-life of these drugs is about two and one half times prolonged. Lincomycin levels are unaffected by peritoneal and haemodialysis.

20.1.8 Fusidic Acid

So little fusidic acid is excreted through the kidneys that no reduction in dosage is required in renal failure. The drug is not significantly removed by haemodialysis.

20.1.9 Nitrofurantoin

In renal failure therapeutically inadequate amounts of nitrofurantoin are found in the urine. Even when there is marginal renal decompensation peripheral neuritis can occur, especially in the elderly. For these reasons nitrofurantoin should not be used when there is any degree of kidney failure.

20.1.10 Nalidixic Acid

Little of this drug appears as therapeutically active nalidixic acid in the urine although there is enough present for the treatment of most sensitive urinary pathogens. Blood levels show only a small rise in uraemic patients; however, the glucuronide of nalidixic acid does accumulate in the urine and although it is not known to be toxic most authorities suggest nalidixic acid should either be avoided in renal failure or given for a very short course only.

20.1.11 Cephalosporins

Because of the decreased likelihood of renal toxicity with cephalothin or cephalexin these drugs are preferred to cephaloridine in uraemic patients. The serum half-lives of both cephaloridine and cephalexin are much prolonged but that of cephalothin only slightly increased. Cephaloridine and frusemide should never be used at the same time. Cephaloridine and cephalothin should not be used concomitantly with aminoglycosides (see section 15.3.5). A watch should be kept for the presence of hyaline casts in the urine when any of the cephalosporins is used in patients with renal failure. Cephalothin is little removed by haemodialysis but when cephalexin is being used 500mg should be given after haemodialysis to keep up the therapeutic level. 1g of cephalothin 8-hourly or 250mg of cephalexin every 24 to 40 hours is recommended for patients with severe renal failure (Garrod et al., 1973).

20.1.12 Peptide Antibiotics

These drugs are both neurotoxic and nephrotoxic and may cause alarming apnoeic episodes if the blood concentration is allowed to rise too high or they are used with curare-like muscle relaxants or aminoglycosides. Special care must therefore be taken when they are used in patients in renal failure. Peak blood levels must be kept well below 10µg/ml and levels of polymyxin B in excess of 5µg/ml make neurotoxicity very likely (Hoeprich, 1970). Curtis and Eastwood (1968) recommend that patients with creatinine clearances of less than 10ml/min should receive 2 to 3mg/kg body weight intravenously every 3 days. A similar dose is recommended at the end of each haemodialysis but is unnecessary after peritoneal dialysis as colistin is cleared poorly by this method.

20.1.13 Aminoglycosides

These drugs are of particular value in the management of the life-threatening infections to which uraemic patients are so vulnerable. They are all potentially nephrotoxic and ototoxic and in renal failure their serum half-lives are considerably prolonged, thus increasing the risk of toxicity. For dosage recommendations the reader is referred to the section on aminoglycosides. Amounts of streptomycin removed by haemodialysis vary and it is advisable to monitor serum levels often. 500mg kanamycin or 80mg gentamicin are recommended as 'top-up' doses after the haemodialysis of patients receiving these drugs (Garrod et al., 1973).

20.1.14 Cycloserine

This drug has been used in the management of recurrent *Esch. coli* urinary tract infections in an adult dose of 250mg 12-hourly. The drug is excreted via the kidneys and the dose must be reduced in renal failure so that the peak serum level remains below 20µg/ml (Gray et al., 1967).

20.1.15 Antituberculosis Drugs (other than streptomycin)

Ogg et al. (1968) showed that isoniazid disappeared slowly from the blood in a patient with severe renal failure. They gave pyridoxine prophylactically and no toxicity was noted. A dose of 150mg isoniazid daily seemed appropriate. Para-aminosalicylate (PAS), which is excreted solely by the kidneys, accumulated in the uraemic patient and doses of 6g between each haemodialysis were given.

Ethambutol is excreted mainly in the urine and the dose should be reduced in renal failure and a careful watch kept for ocular toxicity (Kovnat et al., 1973).

Rifamide does not accumulate in uraemic patients and may be given in normal doses. McGeachie et al. (1970) suggest that this drug could be used for the treatment of staphylococcal infection in patients with chronic renal failure.

20.2 Hepatic Disease

Certain antibacterial drugs are hepatotoxic causing deranged liver function either by hepatocellular injury or by cholestasis. These drugs must be used cautiously when liver function is already compromised. Other drugs, which may or may not be hepatotoxic, are largely metabolised in the liver and so should not be used at all in liver failure or prescribed in reduced dosage if no alternative exists. No description will be given here of the prehepatic haemolytic jaundice sometimes induced by drugs such as sulphonamides, penicillin G, choramphenicol, novobiocin, nitrofurantoin and PAS. Some of these drugs cause jaundice by several different mechanisms. The use of drugs which may harm the liver in the premature baby, or accumulate because of poorly developed hepatic enzymes in the very young, is described elsewhere (see section 21).

20.2.1 Drugs Causing Hepatocellular Damage

Tetracyclines
Fatty change in the hepatocytes of patients treated with tetracyclines is most likely to occur in the course of pregnancy or renal failure, particularly when high intravenous doses are given (Schultz et al., 1963; Lepper et al., 1951). These drugs are best avoided in pregnancy because of their effect on fetal teeth and bone growth (see section 21.4.5).

Oxacillin
This drug may cause fever, vomiting and elevation of the serum transaminase level (Dismukes, 1973) presumably because more of it than the other isoxazolyl penicillins is excreted via the liver.

Sulphonamides

Hepatotoxicity is well documented (Dujovne et al., 1967) and often results from a combination of direct liver cell injury with cholestasis.

Pyrazinamide and Thiacetazone

Both of these antituberculous drugs can cause severe hepatotoxicity.

20.2.2 Drugs Causing Hepatitis-like Reactions

Isoniazid

This drug may rarely cause hepatitis-like liver injury. The light microscopic appearances of a liver biopsy taken from a patient with isoniazid-induced liver disease closely resemble those of viral hepatitis.

Ethionamide

Disturbances of liver function without jaundice or liver cell damage may be caused by ethionamide, especially in diabetic subjects (Moulding and Goldstein, 1962; Phillips and Tashman, 1963; Conn et al., 1964).

Ampicillin and Carbenicillin

Knirsch and Gralla (1970) have reported elevated transaminase levels in patients treated with parenteral ampicillin and carbenicillin but this effect is not thought to indicate hepatotoxicity so much as local muscle irritation at the injection site.

20.2.3 Drugs Causing Cholestasis

Oleandomycin and Erythromycin Estolate

These, but not other forms of erythromycin, can cause cholestasis and hepatitis-like reactions if used for more than 14 days (see section 9.1.6 and 9.2).

Nitrofurantoin

Exacerbation of already existing liver disease was documented by Strauss and Jawetz (1963). Bhagwat and Warren (1969), reporting on one further case, found only 6 proven examples of nitrofurantoin induced hepatotoxicity in the published literature between 1960 and 1969.

20.2.4 Drugs Mainly Metabolised or Detoxicated by the Liver

In general these drugs should be avoided in liver failure or, if it is found essential to use them, prescribed in reduced dosage with careful monitoring of blood levels.

Penicillins

Of the penicillin group, oxacillin is the most likely to cause problems in patients with hepatic failure as it is excreted through the liver more than the other penicillins.

Chloramphenicol

In some patients with advanced cirrhosis Kunin et al. (1959) found that the half-life of active chloramphenicol was prolonged because of slower glucuronidation. Therefore, this drug should not be used in liver failure without dosage reduction and careful serum monitoring.

Tetracyclines

The already mentioned hepatotoxicity of these drugs suggests that they should be used very cautiously, if at all, in liver failure. They are also known to accumulate when hepatic function is poor.

Macrolides

As these drugs tend to reach high levels in severe liver disease, dose reduction is required and serum levels should be monitored if they are to be used.

Novobiocin

If suitable alternatives are available this drug should be avoided in liver disease because it is largely excreted through the bile. Novobiocin should not be used in neonates (section 21.4.7).

Lincomycin and Clindamycin

These drugs are best avoided in severe liver failure, but if used, serum levels should be checked regularly (Kucers and Bennett, 1975).

Fusidic Acid

Little is known about the behaviour of this drug in liver disease.

Nitrofurantoin

Because of the rare but recognised hepatic toxicity of nitrofurantoin (Bhagwat and Warren, 1969) it should probably be avoided in patients with liver failure.

Nalidixic Acid

Although nalidixic acid is largely excreted in the urine, it is mostly in a conjugated, pharmacologically inactive state. Conjugation may not proceed normally when hepatic function is deranged so this drug is not advised in liver failure.

Peptide Antibiotics

As these drugs are little metabolised in the body and are not cleared through the bile, there would appear to be no contraindication to their use in hepatic failure.

Cephalosporins

There appears to be no contraindication to the use of cephalosporins in patients with hepatic dysfunction — with the possible exception of cephaloglycin which is metabolised in the liver before being excreted in the urine.

21. Antibacterial Therapy in Infants and Children

21.1 General Considerations

At no other time in life is the human being more susceptible to serious bacterial infection than in the perinatal period, the premature or low birth weight infant being particularly at risk. The fetus may be infected transplacentally by bacteria such as *Treponema pallidum*, protozoons such as *Toxoplasma gondii* and viruses such as rubella, cytomegalovirus and varicella. Premature rupture of the membranes or a prolonged labour expose the unborn infant to bacterial pathogens from the infected liquor. Later, during his passage through the birth canal, the infant may be contaminated by gonococci, spirochaetes, *Listeria* and other bacteria, *Mycoplasma pneumoniae*, chlamydia and viruses such as *Herpes simplex*.

Even under ideal conditions, the healthy mother delivers her healthy, uncontaminated baby from her bacteriologically sterile uterus into a highly infectious environment. Within a few hours, or days at most, the infant becomes colonised with commensal and pathogenic micro-organisms via the skin, eyes, umbilicus, mouth, respiratory passages, anterior urethra and the female genital tract (Williams, 1974; Davies et al., 1970). The degree to which the baby is invaded by this microbial onslaught depends on several factors. If he is breast fed, alone by his mother at home, he will acclimatise to his microbiological environment more gently than if he is handled by different attendants and bottle fed beside other infants in a hospital nursery. If colonisation proceeds too rapidly or the bacterial invasion is too massive, the neonate's underdeveloped cellular and immune defence mechanisms become overwhelmed and infection results. It is not surprising therefore that antibacterial drugs are the most frequently prescribed therapeutic agents in the newborn period.

If effective antibacterial therapy, without toxicity, is to be given to these vulnerable infants, it is important to have a clear understanding of the pharmacokinetics of drugs in the immature, but rapidly developing, metabolic and excretory processes of the neonate (Yaffe and Back, 1966; Yaffe and Simon, 1970). The prescription of antimicrobial drugs to the newborn — and especially to the premature infant — in doses based purely on body weight or surface area compared with an adult, cannot be too strongly condemned and may account for many of the toxic drug reactions reported in this age group.

Other considerations in the perinatal period and beyond concern antibacterial drugs given to the mother during pregnancy, labour and lactation (Gill and Davis, 1974; Thistlethwaite, 1974). Only that component of a drug which is unbound to maternal plasma proteins can cross the placenta. High lipid solubility and low ionisation at maternal pH favour transfer. Some antibacterial agents may cause dysorganogenesis (8th nerve deafness with aminoglycosides), growth retardation and calcium chelation in bones and teeth (tetracyclines), sensitisation (penicillins and sulphonamides), competition with unconjugated bilirubin for albumin binding sites (novobiocin and sulphonamides), methaemoglobinaemia (sulphonamides), haemolytic anaemia in infants with reduced glucose-6-phosphate dehydrogenase (nalidixic acid, nitrofurantoin, sulphonamides), pyridoxine deficiency and convulsions, rarely, (isoniazid) and again, rarely, Coombs positive haemolytic anaemia (penicillin).

Drugs may also diffuse into breast milk in small amounts, especially if they are lipid soluble, or there is maternal renal insufficiency. Drugs known to be secreted in milk include the penicillins, erythromycin, lincomycin, chloramphenicol, aminoglycosides, novobiocin, sulphonamides, nitrofurantoin and nalidixic acid. Enough may appear in breast milk to sensitise the infant.

Because of his immature immune state the premature infant or neonate may frequently develop serious infections, such as septicaemia or meningitis, with organisms such as Gram-negative bacilli which are regarded as healthy commensals in the gastrointestinal tract of an older patient. Congenital anatomical abnormalities also predispose to infection: pyelonephritis in the obstructed urinary tract, ascending cholangitis in biliary malformations, respiratory infections with unrepaired oesophagotracheal fistulae and meningitis in spina bifida. Septicaemia often results from these infections and in a child with congenital heart disease there is a major risk of bacterial endocarditis. Respiratory viruses — to which an older child may have developed some immunity — invade the susceptible infant, inflame the airways and prepare them for subsequent bacterial invasion. The baby with cystic fibrosis is particularly prone to respiratory infection by staphylococci and *Ps. aeruginosa*. Gastrointestinal invaders include *Esch. coli* which most frequently disrupt gut function in the bottle fed infant who is deprived of the high IgA content in colostrum and breast milk. These *Esch. coli* serotypes seldom induce diarrhoea in older children or adults but in the infant they can cause a prolonged deficiency of enzymes, especially lactase, with consequent malabsorption.

21.2 Dosage

Special precautions must be observed, for the underweight or premature infant especially, and for the full term baby in the first 2 weeks of life, both in the choice of antibacterial agent and the dosage employed. Perinatal doses are in general one half to two thirds that of the dose calculated according to body weight or age (Garrod et al.,

1973a) and will be considered separately for each major antibacterial agent. For the older infant or child, a percentage method based on Leech and Wood (1967) can be used to determine the dose. Hutchison (1974) suggests that a full term infant of 3.2kg requires 12.5% of the average adult dose: a 12-month-old baby weighing 10kg requires 25%: a 7-year-old child weighing 23kg requires 50% and a 12-year-old child of 40kg requires 75% of the average adult dose.

A closely similar method also based on Catzel and propounded by Leech and Wood (1967) recommends that if the adult dose is 1 mg/kg body weight then the dose between 2 weeks and 1 year is 2mg/kg; at 1 to 7 years 1.5mg/kg and at 12 years 1.25mg/kg body weight. Both of these schedules work well in practice.

21.3 Clinical Pharmacology of Antibacterial Drugs in the Premature Infant and Newborn

The fate of antimicrobials in the body depends on their absorption, protein and tissue binding, distribution in different organs and body fluids and on their metabolism in and excretion from the body. Without a clear understanding of these mechanisms, which are often very different in the premature and newborn infant, effective concentrations of antibacterial agents cannot be achieved in the infected body compartments without the risk of serious toxicity (Yaffe and Simon, 1970; Davies et al., 1970). Peak levels of parenterally administered antibacterial drugs are reached almost simultaneously in infants and adults so that problems of absorption do not apply when the drug is given by this route (Yaffe and Simon, 1970). There is some disagreement about the significance of the relative size of body compartments in the infant and adult and whether this should influence antibiotic prescribing (Yaffe and Simon, 1970; Gill and Davis, 1974). Nonetheless, the main problems of dosage in the premature infant relate to protein binding, metabolism, detoxication and excretion of the antimicrobial agents.

21.3.1 Protein Binding

In the presence of jaundice or acidaemia, both bilirubin and hydrogen ions will compete with antibacterial drugs for protein binding sites, making the serum concentration of active unbound drug much higher than normal. Conversely drugs like novobiocin and the long acting sulphonamides bind to plasma proteins so strongly that large amounts of displaced unconjugated bilirubin penetrate into central nervous system tissues and increase the risk of kernicterus.

21.3.2 Metabolism and Detoxication

High antibiotic serum concentrations may occur in premature and newborn infants because of their immature enzyme development. The classical example is the administration of large doses of chloramphenicol to premature infants resulting in the 'grey baby' syndrome. Nyhan (1961) reviewed the features of this syndrome. 2 to 9 days after starting chloramphenicol the infant fails to feed, vomits, sometimes has diarrhoea and develops shallow irregular respirations. Within 12 to 24 hours of onset an ashen grey cyanosis sets in, with hypothermia, flaccidity and death. As the amount of free chloramphenicol in the urine of infants is equivalent to that of adults and as the half-life of the free drug is not prolonged in anuric adults (Kunin et al., 1959) it seems unlikely that the toxic accumulation of free chloramphenicol in premature infants is due to poor renal excretion. It is concluded, therefore, that the toxic serum levels of free chloramphenicol result from the inability of the neonatal liver enzymes to glucuronidate the drug. Fortunately many antibacterial agents are largely excreted unchanged in the urine without significant metabolism being necessary, however, nalidixic acid, like chloramphenicol depends upon glucuronidation and is similarly toxic in the newborn. Very occasionally fetal exposure to drugs *in utero* may induce enzyme activity, hasten drug metabolism in the neonate and lead to serum concentrations that are therapeutically inadequate.

21.3.3 Renal Excretion

Compared with the older child or adult, renal blood flow and glomerular filtration rates are relatively low in the premature baby and even in the full term baby during the first 2 weeks of life. The serum half-life of renally excreted antibacterial agents approaches that found in adults only by the time the infant is a month old, irrespective of the degree of prematurity (Yaffe and Simon, 1970). This finding suggests that the postnatal rather than the gestational age is more important in the clearance of renally excreted antimicrobials. This contrasts with the anatomical observation that new nephrons are produced postnatally in premature infants. Yaffe and Simon (1970) therefore conclude that whilst nephrogenesis is commensurate with gestational age, maturation in terms of antibiotic clearance is independent of gestational age.

21.3.4 Genetic Factors

Infants with certain inherited enzyme defects such as glucose-6-phosphate dehydrogenase deficiency may develop severe haemolysis with drugs such as sulphonamides, nalidixic acid and nitrofurantoin.

21.4 Special Considerations with Individual Drugs

Antibacterial drugs which are contraindicated in the newborn are listed in table X.

Table X. Antibacterial drugs contraindicated in the newborn

Sulphonamides and co-trimoxazole
Tetracyclines
Nalidixic acid and oxolinic acid
Nitrofurantoin
Novobiocin
Lincomycin and clindamycin

21.4.1 Sulphonamides

Despite animal experiments suggesting dysmorphogenicity with long acting sulphonamides, a retrospective study failed to show a similar effect in man (Garrod et al., 1973b). However, sulphonamides cross the placenta with ease and may sensitise the fetus. Sulphamethoxypyridazine, derived transplacentally from the mother, has been shown to circulate in the fetus for days and to be excreted very slowly after birth (Sparr and Pritchard, 1958). Sulphonamides compete with bilirubin for protein binding sites and so increase the risk of kernicterus. In the premature infant whose glucuronyl transferase activity is underdeveloped, the unconjugated bilirubin concentration may be even further increased because that proportion of the sulphonamide dose which would normally be acetylated or converted into glucuronide in the liver of an older individual is not detoxicated. Immature renal function in the perinatal period also tends to prolong the serum half-life of the drug. Sulphonamides, therefore, should be avoided in the neonatal period. Kucers and Bennett (1975a) recommend that daily doses of up to 150mg/kg/body weight can be safely given to the older infant or child who is severely infected. A further hazard in children is the association between the Stevens-Johnson syndrome and long acting sulphonamides.

21.4.2 The Penicillins

Riley (1970) has reviewed the literature on penicillin and cephalosporin therapy in paediatric practice.

Penicillin G
The renal clearance of penicillin G in premature and newborn infants is only 17% of the clearance value in older children when calculated for surface area and 34% when corrected for body weight (Barnett et al., 1949). Very high serum concentrations of penicillin may therefore be attained in the perinatal period. McCracken et al. (1973) showed that a total daily dose of 50,000 units of penicillin G/kg body weight divided into 8 or 12 hourly injections in neonates produced serum levels more than adequate for treating systemic infections caused by sensitive bacteria. A single daily dose of 50,000 units of procaine penicillin G was adequate for treating minor

Table XI. Suggested doses of antibacterial drugs in the newborn

Drug	Route	Total daily dose units or mg/kg body weight	Number of doses in 24hrs	Comment
Penicillins				
Penicillin G	im/iv	50,000-100,000 units	4	
Penicillin V	oral	62.5-125mg	4	
Methicillin	im	100mg	4	
Cloxacillin	oral	62.5mg	4	
	im/iv	50-100mg	4	
Ampicillin	oral	62.5mg	4	
	im/iv	50-100mg	4	
Carbenicillin	im/iv	100mg initially then 75mg till 4 days old then 100mg thereafter	4	For infants weighing over 2kg
	im/iv	100mg initially then 75mg till 7 days old then 100mg thereafter	3	For infants weighing under 2kg
			4	
Chloramphenicol	oral/im	15-25mg	4	May be doubled for first 48 hours in meningitis in full term babies. Only use in pre-term if no other suitable drug available and keep to the smaller dose for the first 4 weeks of life.
Erythromycin	oral	25-50mg	4	
	iv	12.5-25mg	2	
Fusidic acid	oral/iv	20mg	4	Caution in the pre-term infant till more data available.

Cepahlosporins			
Cephaloridine ⎫	im/iv	30mg	4
Cephalothin ⎬			
Cephalexin	oral	30mg	4
Peptide antibiotics			
Colistin sulphomethate	im	3-5mg (37,500-62,500 units)	3	Intrathecal colistin methosulphate may be given in a single daily dose of 0.04mg/kg/day (500 units/kg/day) using a preparation without cinchocaine.
Aminoglycosides				Serum levels *must* be monitored. The larger doses quoted are for full term babies after the first 48 hours of life. The smaller doses should be adhered to in pre-term babies for the first 7 days of life and in full term for the first 48 hours of life.
Streptomycin	im	20-30mg	2	Streptomycin may be given intrathecally to the newborn in a single *total* daily dose of 1mg.
Kanamycin	im	7.5-10mg	2	Kanamycin may be given intrathecally to the newborn in a single *total* daily dose of 2-3mg.
Gentamicin	im/iv	3.0-5mg	2	Gentamicin may be given intrathecally to the newborn in a single *total* daily dose of 1-2mg.
Tobramycin	im	4mg	2	

infections with sensitive organisms and for congenital syphilis. Reports of sterile abscesses following injections of procaine penicillin rather militate against its use in the newborn and serious infections should be treated with penicillin G alone.

Ampicillin

Yaffe and Simon (1970) studied the mean serum half-life of ampicillin in premature infants after an intramuscular dose of 10mg/kg body weight. It was 4 hours in 9 infants 2 to 7 days old and 1.6 hours in 9 who were 31 to 68 days of age, compared with a serum half-life in the adult of 1.3 to 1.5 hours. Kaplan et al. (1974) suggest that premature infants in the first month of life should receive 100mg/kg body weight daily, divided in 2 doses, given every 12 hours. For severe infections such as septicaemia, ampicillin should be given in combination with kanamycin or gentamicin until the sensitivity of the organism is known. In older children doses are calculated by age or body weight.

Methicillin

Yaffe and Simon (1970) showed that after a 20mg/kg body weight intramuscular injection the serum level of methicillin was 1.8μg/ml in infants less than 1 week old, but it was undetectable in older infants, suggesting that renal clearance approached the adult level a week or two after birth. Doses of 25 to 50mg/kg body weight daily given as 2 doses every 12 hours are sufficient for premature babies.

Isoxazolyl Penicillins

As for methicillin, Axline et al. (1967) suggest 25 to 50mg/kg body weight daily, given in 2 doses 12-hourly, for premature babies requiring treatment with an isoxazolyl penicillin. Higher doses are recommended for mature neonates after the first two weeks of life (see table XI).

Carbenicillin

Nelson and McCracken (1973) have devised a dosage schedule which should assure therapeutic serum concentrations in neonates: 100mg/kg body weight as an initial dose followed by 75mg/kg body weight in doses at 8-hourly intervals for 7 days for infants less than 2kg and at 6-hourly intervals until 4 days of age for infants weighing more than 2kg. Thereafter a dose of 100mg/kg body weight every 6 hours is satisfactory in both weight groups. Carbenicillin in these doses combined with gentamicin was as effective as a combination of ampicillin and gentamicin in the management of severely infected neonates.

21.4.3 Co-trimoxazole

Co-trimoxazole should not be given to premature infants or neonates until more data are available. Roy (1971) gave trimethoprim in a dose of 8 to 10mg/kg body

weight per day and sulphamethoxazole 40 to 50mg/kg body weight per day to neonates. One infant 3 weeks old, desperately ill with postoperative septicaemia, died
after treatment with co-trimoxazole and a pancytopenia, possibly related to drug
therapy, was noted. Another infant of 7 days survived an *Esch. coli* meningitis and
only a marginal transient neutropenia was found after co-trimoxazole treatment. The
place of trimethoprim alone in the management of coliform meningitis is still to be
evaluated but could be promising as some CSF penetration of the drug occurs in
meningitis (Garrod et al., 1973c).

21.4.4 Chloramphenicol

The pharmacokinetics of chloramphenicol in the neonatal period have been
described by Nyhan (1961) [see section 21.3.2]. In 1959 Burns et al. reported a 60%
mortality amongst 61 premature babies given chloramphenicol in doses ranging from
100 to 165mg/kg body weight daily. Of 15 premature infants receiving approximately 150mg/kg body weight daily prophylactically 6 died compared with only 2
in a control group of 16 untreated infants (Lambdin et al., 1960). Providing serum
levels of active chloramphenicol do not exceed 20µg/ml the 'grey baby' syndrome
should not occur (Weiss et al., 1960; Yaffe, 1965), but as doses as low as 25mg/kg
body weight per day may be associated with toxic serum levels in the newborn,
monitoring is very important. Chloramphenicol should not be used unless no suitable
alternative is available. Cocke et al. (1966) reported optic neuritis in an 18-week-old
child which was attributed to prolonged chloramphenicol treatment of cystic fibrosis.
Huang et al. (1966) report similar toxicity in 9 of 33 patients also treated for cystic
fibrosis with long term chloramphenicol.

21.4.5 Tetracyclines

The main disadvantage of the use of tetracyclines in infants and children is their
deposition in teeth and bones. Kucers and Bennett (1975b) have reviewed this subject
admirably. The drugs cross the placenta and are deposited in the developing
deciduous teeth of the fetus, often causing unsightly discoloration. The secondary
dentition may be permanently affected if children under the age of 7 years are
given tetracyclines. If one of these drugs must be given at this vulnerable age,
either doxycycline or oxytetracycline should be used as they cause less discoloration. Courses should be limited to 7 days. It is not definitely known yet whether
the affected teeth are defective or only discolored. Cohlan et al. (1963) demonstrated temporary inhibition of the bone growth of infants given tetracycline
but permanent changes in the human bone structure have so far not been reported.

21.4.6 Macrolides

Erythromycin appears safe in neonates, 40mg/kg body weight daily of the estolate being given to 26 premature infants without clinical signs of toxicity or elevation of serum enzymes (Burns and Hodgman, 1963). Information about the other macrolides in the newborn period is not available.

21.4.7 Novobiocin

This drug is concentrated in the liver and strongly protein bound so that by displacement of bilirubin, kernicterus may be caused. A three-fold rise in neonatal bilirubinaemia was found by Sutherland and Keller (1961) when using novobiocin. This drug is therefore absolutely contraindicated in the first month of life.

21.4.8 Lincomycin and Clindamycin

Both drugs cross the placenta and the concentrations in milk are similar to the maternal serum level (Kucers and Bennett, 1975c). Because of the variable degree of protein binding it would seem unwise to use these drugs in the neonate, especially in the presence of jaundice, until more data are available.

21.4.9 Fusidic Acid

Little is known about the effect of this drug on the newborn but caution should be exercised if it is used in the perinatal period because of its high degree of protein binding. Little fusidic acid is excreted in the urine or faeces and it is presumed that the drug is metabolised in the body; thus it is possible that immature neonatal enzyme systems might not be adequate. Thistlethwaite (1974) recommends 20 to 40mg/kg body weight per day either orally or parenterally. Liddy (1973) gave intravenous fusidic acid as diethanolamine fusidate to 5 newborn infants in a dose of 20mg/kg body weight in 24 hours without observing local or systemic toxicity.

21.4.10 Nitrofurantoin

Nitrofurantoin like nalidixic acid should not be used in the neonatal period because immature enzyme systems in the liver and erythrocytes of the newborn cannot detoxify the drug and dangerous serum levels result; see section 12 (Finegold and Ziment, 1968).

21.4.11 Nalidixic Acid

This drug which is excreted poorly in the urine, and which is highly plasma bound, should not be used in the premature infant or neonate. Anderson (1971) who described papilloedema and bilateral 6th nerve palsy in a 5-year-old girl treated with nalidixic acid, also refers to several other previous associations between nalidixic acid therapy and intracranial hypertension in young patients.

21.4.12 Cephalosporins

In neonates a single dose of cephaloridine 15mg/kg body weight per day gives higher and more prolonged serum levels than is obtained with a single dose of 1g in the adult (Kucers and Bennett, 1975d). Burland and Simpson (1967) suggest 15mg/kg body weight in 2 or 3 doses during the day for the newborn and a minimum dosage of 15mg/kg body weight twice daily in premature babies. For severe infections cephalothin 25mg/kg body weight may be given safely 4 to 6 hourly, although one half to one third of this dose is usually sufficient (Wise, 1973). Although doses of cephalexin up to 100mg/kg body weight per day have been used without toxicity in the newborn, the slower excretion of this drug permits doses of 25 to 50mg/kg body weight per day to be adequate therapy for the newborn (Marget, 1971).

21.4.13 Polypeptide Antibiotics

Yaffe and Simon (1970) studied the serum half-life of colistin sulphomethate in premature infants after a single intramuscular dose of 5mg/kg body weight. It was 2.6 hours in infants 4 days old, and 2.3 hours in infants of 12 to 51 days of age, compared with a mean serum half-life of 2 to 3 hours in the older children and adults. It seemed that the serum half-life did not decline with increasing postnatal age and Yaffe and Simon (1970) suggest that the excretion of colistin might depend on mechanisms other than glomerular filtration in the premature infant. A dose of between 3 and 5mg/kg body weight per day therefore seems adequate for neonates, given either intravenously or intramuscularly. For meningitis caused by Gram-negative bacilli colistin sulphomethate may be given in a dose of 0.04mg/kg body weight per day, by the intrathecal route, using a preparation which does *not* contain cinchocaine.

21.4.14 Aminoglycosides

High levels of streptomycin have been shown in fetal CSF leading to 8th nerve damage in the offspring of mothers given streptomycin in pregnancy. Similarly, transplacentally mediated kanamycin ototoxicity has been recorded (Thistlethwaite, 1974). The dangers of ototoxicity and nephrotoxicity are increased in the premature and newborn whose kidney function is immature. The serum half-life of aminoglycosides is prolonged in the first week of life. So far as gentamicin is concerned, the half-life is more dependent on postnatal than post gestational age (Yaffe and Simon, 1970). Doses must be reduced, therefore, in full term as well as premature babies in the first few days of life. Aminoglycoside dosage regimens appropriate to the newborn are set out in table XI.

Opinions differ about the degree of protein binding of aminoglycosides and the consequent risk of kernicterus but as these drugs can be life saving in neonatal septicaemia, they should be used and the serum levels carefully monitored. For the long term treatment of tuberculosis in children the recommended dose of streptomycin is 20mg/kg body weight daily.

21.4.15 Hexachlorophane

This substance is incorporated in dusting powders and emulsions for application to the hands of attendants and the skin of newborn babies in an attempt to reduce staphylococcal infection. Animal experiments show that it is toxic to the myelin of the CNS. Powell et al. (1973) reported a number of infants with myelinopathy proven at autopsy which they attributed to the use of hexachlorophane. Babies most at risk are premature or low birth weight infants who receive numerous applications of hexachlorophane, particularly if they have skin rashes or sepsis, abrasions, wounds or are allowed to ingest hexachlorophane from too close application to the mouth. Alder et al. (1972) showed significant amounts of hexachlorophane in the cord blood of healthy infants treated with the substance, but as the levels, with one possible exception, were well below those considered toxic for animals they advocate the continued use of this preparation. Used carefully according to the manufacturers' instructions, the benefits accruing from the use of hexachlorophane in reducing staphylococcal sepsis in a nursery far outweigh the risks.

21.5 Specific Infections in Infants

21.5.1 Congenital Syphilis

For an infant of normal body weight a 14 day course of penicillin G in a dose of 50,000 units 6-hourly is recommended.

21.5.2 Gonococcal Ophthalmia

A combination of drops containing 2500 units of penicillin per ml frequently instilled into both conjunctival sacs until the discharge clears, together with a week's course of penicillin G 50,000 units 6-hourly is recommended, followed by a further week's treatment with oral penicillin V.

21.5.3 Staphylococcal Infections

The incidence of these may be reduced by the judicious use of hexachlorophane but they still constitute a menace in the newborn nursery. Sites of predilection for staphylococci are the skin, conjunctivae, nail-folds, umbilicus, breast and more seriously the lungs, meninges and bones. Any of these infections may be associated with staphylococcal septicaemia. Treatment with one of the isoxazolyl penicillins, or if the organism is sensitive with erythromycin, is preferable in the premature infant to treatment with lincomycin or fusidic acid — at least until more data are available for these latter 2 drugs. After the first 2 weeks of life any of the above drugs is suitable. Staphylococcal conjunctivitis will usually respond to frequent instillation of 0.5 % chloramphenicol eye drops.

21.5.4 Gram-negative Bacillary Septicaemia

As a result of rapid bacterial colonisation and poor cellular and humoral immunity, bacteraemia with *Esch. coli, Proteus* spp. *Klebsiella, Ps. aeruginosa* and other Gram-negative bacilli is common in premature and newborn infants. Infection may present with signs as insignificant as listlessness, failure to gain weight, diarrhoea (often with abdominal distension) or jaundice. On the earliest suspicion cultures of blood, urine and CSF must be taken and antibacterial treatment begun. When septicaemia is diagnosed, but the organism responsible is still unknown, gentamicin in combination with cloxacillin is appropriate. Once the result of culture and sensitivity is known one of the antibiotics can usually be withdrawn and treatment continued for 10 to 14 days with a single drug.

21.5.5 Meningitis in Children

In the newborn Gram-negative bacilli cause meningitis far more commonly than do meningococci and pneumococci. Meningitis is usually secondary to septicaemia. The premature, low birth weight infant delivered after a long labour is particularly prone to infection. Signs of meningeal irritation in these infants may be absent and, as with septicaemia, failure to feed, vomiting, diarrhoea, jaundice, irritability or convulsions should alert the paediatrician to take blood and CSF for cultures urgently. The CSF in coliform meningitis may look normal or have a few erythrocytes present, yet the culture may be positive (Heckmatt, 1976). The laboratory should be asked to provide sensitivity patterns for a wide range of antibacterial drugs, including the aminoglycosides, penicillins, cephalosporins, chloramphenicol and polymyxin. The most common Gram-negative organisms are *Esch. coli,* coliforms, klebsiella, aerobacter, flavobacteriae, *Cloaca* spp., *Ps. aeruginosa* and, rarely, *H. influenzae.* Initial treatment should be given with gentamicin, which includes most strains of pseudomonas in its antibacterial range, in a parenteral dose of 5 mg/kg body weight per day, supplemented by 1mg of gentamicin daily by the intrathecal route. Combined therapy with a penicillin is often advocated initially. Chloramphenicol has the major advantage of crossing the blood brain barrier but the disadvantage of toxicity in the very young. If used, the maximum permitted dose for a full term infant is 25mg/kg body weight per day, and it should not be used in the premature infant unless a suitable alternative is unavailable (see section 21.4.4). Heckmatt (1976) recommends the combination of chloramphenicol and gentamicin for coliform meningitis in the newborn. The polypeptide drugs can be used in the management of neonatal meningitis as an alternative to gentamicin. Parenteral colistin methosulphate is given in a dose of 3 to 5mg/kg body weight per day in divided doses with a single daily intrathecal injection of colistin in a dose not exceeding 0.04mg/kg body weight per day, using a preparation without cinchocaine (see section 21.4.13).

Penicillin Sensitive Meningitis

If the organism isolated is penicillin sensitive, for example *Listeria monocytogenes*, penicillin G should replace the more toxic drugs. In later infancy and childhood, *N. meningitidis* and *Str. pneumoniae* may be successfully treated with penicillin G.

Haemophilus influenzae Meningitis

This is the most common cause of childhood meningitis in the USA outside the neonatal period; in the UK meningococci predominate. *H. influenzae* meningitis may occur at any age, although it is less frequent in adults. The symptoms are less abrupt than those found in meningococcal or pneumococcal meningitis. In infants signs of meningeal irritation may be minimal or absent and the child fully conscious despite a grossly purulent CSF. The choice of antibiotics is between chloramphenicol and ampicillin. Chloramphenicol sodium succinate is given in a dose of 25mg/kg body weight per day to mature neonates and 75mg/kg body weight per day as 6-hourly injections in older children. When clinical improvement is noted the patient may be placed on oral treatment with chloramphenicol in a dose of 100mg/kg body weight per day; this should be continued for at least 10 days but not longer than 14.

Ampicillin does not cross the blood brain barrier as well as chloramphenicol and some *H. influenzae* produce β-lactamase (see section 4.4.1). Nevertheless given in high concentrations of 150mg/kg body weight per day sensitive *H. influenzae* meningitis may be treated successfully with ampicillin. The fears of inducing deafness by these high doses seem less well substantiated than was originally thought (Dahnsjo et al., 1976). Less good alternatives to chloramphenicol and ampicillin are the aminoglcyoside drugs. They have the disadvantage of poor CSF penetration so that intrathecal therapy is required. Co-trimoxazole may possibly be used in the older child in the future because of the good penetration of trimethoprim into CSF.

21.5.6 Urinary Infection

Sulphonamides, nalidixic acid and nitrofurantoin should not be used in the neonate. Ampicillin, or one of the cephalosporins or aminoglycosides may be required depending on the sensitivity of the organisms. Frequent blood culturing is necessary to detect bacteraemia and, if the infant is very ill, frequent monitoring of blood levels of these drugs is mandatory.

21.5.7 Gastroenteritis

The temptation to treat neonatal diarrhoea with antibacterial agents must be resisted unless it is strongly suspected that the diarrhoea is a symptom of a more serious process, such as septicaemia. There is no good evidence to show that pathogenic *Esch. coli* gastroenteritis is improved by antibiotics, nor that the elimination of the organisms from the faeces is hastened. Some workers suggest, however, that antibacterial drugs should be used to prevent the spread of infection in a nursery; thus it seems unwise for antibacterial drugs to be employed unless there is clinical or laboratory evidence of septicaemia. It is also doubtful if salmonella or shigella infections are ameliorated by antibiotics unless septicaemia is present.

21.5.8 Cystic Fibrosis

Respiratory infections are common in cystic fibrosis. Precipitin studies in patients with this disease compared with controls showed a marked preponderance of *Staph. pyogenes, Ps. aeruginosa* and *H. influenzae* (Burns and May, 1968). Acute exacerbations of respiratory infection must be appropriately treated with antibacterial drugs such as isoxazolyl penicillins and aminoglycosides, mucolytics and physiotherapy. In between acute attacks, long term treatment with antistaphylococcal drugs such as cloxacillin has its advocates (Mearns, 1974), although most paediatricians, aware of the risk of colonisation with *Ps. aeruginosa* or the development of resistance by the staphylococci, would only treat when infection was reasonably certain (McCrae, 1974; Raeburn, 1976).

21.5.9 Whooping Cough

Bordetella pertussis is sensitive to a number of antibiotics but after a clinical attack of whooping cough has started there is nothing to be gained by giving antibacterial treatment unless a secondary bacterial broncho-pneumonia sets in. Recently prophylactic erythromycin (Altemeier and Ayoub, 1977) has been shown to protect non-immunised infants in contact with pertussis from developing the disease. In the very young this drug is better tolerated so it should be used in preference to its rival co-trimoxazole.

22. Antibacterial Therapy in the Elderly

Before dealing with the more common infections encountered in the elderly, the principles which should guide the prescribing of antibacterials for this group of patients will be discussed.

22.1 General Principles

Information relating to the absorption, distribution and elimination of antibacterial agents is usually obtained from volunteer studies in healthy young adults rather than patients. Studies in the elderly are rare. Antibacterial therapy in this age group requires more care than it is often accorded. Failure of therapy, or toxicity, may be encountered because of failure to absorb or excrete antibacterial drugs in the same way as do younger patients. Little is known of the absorption of drugs in the elderly: however it is recognised that deficient absorption may be caused by the simultaneous administration of other drugs, for example the defective absorption of tetracyclines when given with oral iron or antacid mixtures. Interactions with other drugs may occur after absorption: potent diuretics, such as frusemide, may enhance the ototoxicity of the aminoglycosides and the nephrotoxicity of cephaloridine (see section 13.1.5); co-trimoxazole may induce toxicity with warfarin or sulphonylureas (see section 2.7); co-trimoxazole may interfere with folate metabolism and the response to haematinics in the elderly in whom folate deficiency is common (see section 6.7.1).

Deterioration of renal function in the elderly may lead to accumulation of antibacterial agents with an associated risk of toxicity. Equally, renal excretion may be sufficiently poor as to lead to subinhibitory urine levels, treatment failure and possibly to the emergence of resistant strains. Elderly patients with apparently normal renal function may excrete penicillins at a slower rate than their younger counterparts, with similar resultant problems.

These examples illustrate the necessity of considering the patient with his or her concomitant diseases as a whole, rather than as an infective problem which at first sight may seem to require merely the prescription of 'an antibiotic'.

22.2 Urinary Tract Infection

Urinary tract infection (UTI) poses special problems in the elderly. Asymptomatic bacteriuria (ASB) is present in up to 30% of elderly women and, in the majority, is not associated with major underlying pathology. Usually no treatment is required. However, UTI may be symptomatic of genital prolapse and occasionally of stones, diverticulae, other bladder disorders or genitourinary cancer.

Symptoms of UTI may be minimal, and commonly only frequency or incontinence of recent onset may point to the diagnosis. These symptoms may also present in elderly males, as may ASB, both being commonly associated with prostatic disease. UTI is a common problem following stroke. Other presentations may include pyrexia of uncertain origin, in which at least 2 urine specimens should be examined routinely, and haematuria which, even if found to be associated with UTI, requires further investigation to exclude malignancy.

22.2.1 Indications for Treatment of Proven UTI

1) Systemic illness with fever, especially if associated with positive blood cultures.
2) Recent onset of urinary incontinence or retention; these are often relieved by prompt chemotherapy.
3) ASB in patients with a known predisposition to systemic infection, e.g. diabetes, stone disease. hydronephrosis.
4) Symptoms which disturb the patient's wellbeing (not that of her medical attendants).

Bacteriuria in the elderly, unless causing symptoms or reflecting underlying pathology, should be tolerated and not treated. Ascending infection is unlikely to occur and the presence of uncomplicated ASB is not associated with deterioration in renal function. If therapy is used unnecessarily, the infection will almost certainly recur, bacterial resistance may be induced, and side effects may be encountered. Management of infection in catheterised patients has been discussed elsewhere (see section 25.1.2).

22.2.2 Drugs of Choice in UTI

UTI in the elderly, as in younger patients, will be caused by *Esch. coli, P. mirabilis,* staphylococci and *Str. faecalis,* infection with such organisms as *Ps. aeruginosa, Klebsiella aerogenes* and indole positive *Proteus* spp. being less common, and suggestive of underlying pathology. Treatment in the majority of cases will be governed by sensitivity tests. In general this will allow a choice of agent, the least toxic of which should always be chosen. Some drugs are best avoided in the elderly, for example nitrofurantoin, which may cause peripheral neuropathy in patients with diminishing renal function, tetracyclines, which may exacerbate existing renal insufficiency, and oral cephalosporins which are associated with distressing candidal superinfection.

Broad spectrum penicillins, for example amoxycillin, the recently introduced mecillinam, and nalidixic acid are effective and relatively free from side effects. Co-trimoxazole should be used with caution in potentially folate deficient subjects. Carbenicillin esters, such as carfecillin and carindacillin, have been implicated in the production of carbenicillin resistance and should be reserved for *Ps. aeruginosa* bacteriuria only.

In systemic infection injectable cephalosporins such as cephaloridine and cephalothin, or aminoglycosides are the drugs of choice, but potential toxicity must be considered. If the organism is known to be sensitive to ampicillin this drug, or amoxycillin, should be used parenterally. Neither should be used as first choice agents on a 'best guess' basis as resistance amongst *Esch. coli* is of the order of 50%.

Treatment of UTI is not complete until post-treatment urine cultures have been shown to be sterile.

22.3 Chest Infection

Pneumonia is common in the elderly, and should always be considered in patients who suddenly become ill and confused. Pyrexia is usual but not invariable and the patient may become extremely ill before chest signs develop. Tachypnoea and intercostal recession are valuable early signs. The main clinical syndromes are fairly clear-cut and are associated with a predictable range of organisms.

Lobar pneumonia, hypostatic pneumonia and pneumonia following hypothermia, are almost always caused by the pneumococcus, and the drug of choice is benzylpenicillin, in a dose of 250,000 units 6 to 8 hourly. It should be continued for 3 to 4 days followed by a 1 week course of phenoxymethyl penicillin.

Aspiration pneumonia is caused by upper respiratory tract commensals, including pneumococci, *Neisseria* spp. and oral anaerobes. These organisms are sensitive to benzylpenicillin which therefore is the drug of choice. Some cases of aspirational lung abscess are associated with *Bacteroides fragilis,* in which event metronidazole 400 to 600mg 8-hourly by mouth, or clindamycin 300 to 600mg 8-hourly by mouth, should be added to the treatment regimen.

Post-viral pneumonia, for example, that occurs after influenza, may be caused by pneumococci or by *Staph. aureus* and requires a drug effective against both organisms. The drug of first choice is cloxacillin, in a dosage of 500mg 6-hourly parenterally for up to 1 week, followed by a further 1 week course of oral flucloxacillin 250mg 6-hourly.

Pneumonia in bronchitic patients may be due to either the pneumococcus or *H. influenzae,* and the patient should be treated with ampicillin or amoxycillin, 500mg 6-hourly, the route of administration being determined by the severity of the illness.

Further help in assessment of the invading pathogen may be gained from the chest x-ray, lobar shadowing indicating pneumococcal disease, widespread ill-defined opacities being consistent with staphylococcal or *H. influenzae* bronchopneumonia (and, rarely, tuberculous bronchopneumonia), and granular 'ground glass' opacification indicating 'atypical pneumonia' which will respond to tetracycline.

In patients with penicillin allergy, pneumococcal and *H. influenzae* pneumonia may be treated with co-trimoxazole and staphylococcal pneumonia with clindamycin. Cephalosporins are disappointing in chest infection and are best avoided.

22.4 Skin and Soft Tissue Infections

These infections may be conveniently classified according to the level at which they occur in the skin and subcutaneous tissue. They are almost always due to staphylococcal or β-haemolytic streptococcal infection.

22.4.1 Impetigo

This may occur as a primary event (impetigo contagiosa), or as secondary infection complicating areas of minor tissue injury, for example, eczema, varicose changes, or skin ulcers. It is usually due to *Staph. aureus* and responds to local cleansing followed by the topical application of 3% tetracycline cream. Antibiotic creams containing fusidic acid should be avoided as their use may lead to staphylococcal resistance to this valuable drug. Impetigo should be distinguished from intertrigo in which a mixed bacterial and yeast infection may occur in areas of skin opposition in the obese. This condition responds well to local cleansing and the use of topical antibiotics is unnecessary and may encourage yeast overgrowth.

22.4.2 Erysipelas

Erysipelas is a severe, rapidly spreading infection of the dermis caused by the entry of β-haemolytic streptococci through a break in the skin. It is confined to the skin but may be complicated by bacteraemia which is rapidly fatal. Erysipelas commonly occurs on the face, where it may be complicated by cavernous sinus thrombosis. Treatment with benzylpenicillin is rapidly effective.

22.4.3 Cellulitis

A deep spreading subcutaneous infection, cellulitis is classically caused by *Staph. aureus*, but nowadays is commonly due to a mixture of this organism and the β-haemolytic streptococcus. Secondary bacteraemia is common. It frequently arises from skin ulcers, whether these be due to ischaemia, diabetes, varicosities or pressure sores. Therapy should always be directed to *Staph. aureus* and cloxacillin is the drug of choice. Erythromycin is a suitable alternative in less severe cases but if parenteral therapy is required in a penicillin sensitive patient clindamycin is preferable.

22.4.4 Lymphangitis

This is an ascending infection of the lymphatic vessels due to the β-haemolytic streptococcus. It arises in a focal area of skin sepsis and in hospitalised patients commonly begins at infected intravenous infusion sites (see section 25.1.1). Benzylpenicillin, combined with the removal of any infected foreign body, is highly effective.

22.4.5 Bedsores

These, unfortunately, are common in the elderly and arise from ischaemic skin necrosis following pressure on the sacral areas, heels and other parts on which the patient has lain. Although not primarily infective in nature, colonisation with skin and bowel commensals rapidly supervenes. The organisms are commonly a mixture of staphylococci, *Str. faecalis* and coliforms and are present in a saprophytic role, in many cases causing no invasive illness. Treatment with antibiotics, either systemically or topically, is not indicated: it is unlikely to do more than reduce the numbers of bacteria, which will return as soon as therapy is stopped; it may encourage the selection of resistant bacteria, such as *Ps. aeruginosa,* and it may cause unnecessary side effects. The use of multiple-antibiotic sprays is to be condemned. The situation is entirely changed if tissue invasion occurs. This event is likely to be due to the organisms encountered in any other form of cellulitis and appropriate therapy should be instituted.

23. Antibacterial Drugs in Obstetrics and Gynaecology

23.1 Obstetrics

Since the thalidomide disaster in the 1950's there has been an increasing awareness of the possible intrauterine effects of drugs, especially those taken in the early months of pregnancy. For this reason many pregnant women will be reluctant to take drugs, and their fears must be alleviated before any therapy is prescribed. However, circumstances will arise when antibacterial drugs will be required. At the outset, it should be explained to the patient, that the drug chosen has been shown clearly to have no specific effects on the fetus, either in animal experiments or in human experience.

23.1.1 Bacteriuria of Pregnancy

Bacteriuria is now well recognised, and it is known that even if it is asymptomatic in the early months of pregnancy, if left untreated about half the patients will develop acute urinary tract infections, and some will develop acute pyelonephritis, with or without septicaemia. Thus, treatment for asymptomatic bacteriuria of pregnancy should be instituted with an antibacterial drug which is effective against the causative organism, but safe as far as the fetus is concerned. Since most of the infections will be caused by *Esch. coli,* it can be clearly stated to the patient that certain antimicrobial drugs will eradicate the infection without harm to herself or her baby. In over 20 years of experience, the author has found cycloserine to be the safest and the most effective antibacterial drug in this context. A dose of 250mg twice daily for 10 days will be effective in over 95% of cases. Some would be satisfied with a straight forward, short term eradicative course, to be repeated if bacteriuria recurs later in the pregnancy; however, cycloserine can be taken continuously in a suppressive dose of 250mg on alternate nights, throughout the pregnancy and into the puerperium, without ill effect on the fetus.

Other antibacterial drugs which can be safely administered during pregnancy are the penicillins (in the absence of a history of patient allergy) the cephalosporins and erythromycin. There are contraindications to the sulphonamides, the tetracyclines and the aminoglycosides, all of which may adversely affect the fetus. The tetracyclines are known to cause discoloration of the primary teeth and the sulphonamides, either alone or in combination with trimethoprim, can cause toxicity of the maternal host thus endangering the fetus (see section 6.7.1). The aminoglycosides can cross the placental barrier and are potentially toxic to the developing 8th nerve nucleus in the fetus.

With the exception of asymptomatic bacteriuria the pregnant woman, in general terms, is usually very healthy. The subject of urinary tract infection in females has been reviewed previously (Murdoch, 1963) and there is little to add to this literature, except that there may be a little less emphasis on the dangers of giving antibacterials to pregnant women. It can be concluded that the common infective illnesses due to bacteria, which might arise during pregnancy, can be effectively treated by appropriate antibacterial drugs which have no adverse effect on the developing child. The prospective mother should be reassured in this respect and her fears allayed by the clinician in charge.

23.2 Gynaecology

Infection of the genital tract in the female is still common but its morbidity and mortality has greatly reduced in the past 30 or so years. Nevertheless, chronic ill health as a result of low grade pelvic sepsis still presents a diagnostic and therapeutic challenge. It is not the purpose of this review to enumerate all the gynaecological pathology, but to make a statement on general principles in relation to genital infection. Antibacterial drugs in the management of gynaecological infection may prove to be quite ineffective unless obvious surgical defects have been previously corrected. The opinion of an expert gynaecologist as well as that of the laboratory worker, should always be sought before antibacterial therapy is instituted as a coordinated approach is essential for the most effective results.

23.2.1 Venereal Disease

Venereal infection in the female is prevalent and is very often unsuspected by the patient herself. There may be no obvious discharge, or one which is disregarded, and only proper evaluation of the bacteriology of high vaginal swabs will elucidate the presence of such common entities as gonococcal infection and trichomonal infestation. Penicillin remains the best treatment for gonococcal infection, whether it be acute or chronic.

23.2.2 Salpingitis

It should be recalled that acute salpingitis may be caused by mixed organisms — Gram-positive, Gram-negative and anaerobic, thus effective treatment may have to be instituted 'blind' on this assumption. The combination of erythromycin or lincomycin, with gentamicin or tobramycin should be effective.

23.2.3 Puerperal Sepsis

Puerperal sepsis is now fortunately rare, but occasionally acute streptococcal or staphyloccal pelvic sepsis may follow delivery, and here treatment with benzylpenicillin in high dosage should be instituted. If the patient has been delivered in hospital it should be suspected that the staphylococcus is penicillinase producing, and flucloxacillin should be added to the regimen. If the patient is allergic to the penicillins, a cephalosporin should be administered: cephradine can be given first systemically and later by mouth. If *Clostridium welchii* has been shown to be the cause, high doses of benzylpenicillin should be given with a cephalosporin as an alternative.

23.2.4 Tuberculous Salpingitis

Chronic inflammatory diseases of the pelvis which fail to respond to the above regimens, should always be a reason for suspecting a tuberculous background. Tuberculous salpingitis is by no means eradicated from the earth, and a thorough search should be made for the organisms, not only in the genital tract, but in the lungs and urinary tract as well.

23.2.5 Acute Pelvic Peritonitis

This may complicate various pathologies within the lower abdomen, and it should be concluded that the organisms involved will again be a mixture of Gram-positive, Gram-negative and anaerobic species. If an aminoglycoside antibiotic is given prior to general anaesthesia, the anaesthetist should be informed, in order to avoid potentiation of the effect of curare-like substances, which may be used in the course of the anaesthesia.

24. Surgical Infections

This section deals with prophylaxis of infection and pyrexia following surgery. Anaerobic infection, including tetanus and clostridial myonecrosis, and infections associated with foreign bodies have been discussed elsewhere (see sections 19 and 25).

24.1 Prophylaxis of Surgical Infection

In the past many patients have suffered as a result of prophylaxis rather than gaining by its use. For example, broad spectrum antibiotic prophylaxis for bowel surgery has predisposed to severe opportunistic infection, such as staphylococcal entercolitis, without significantly reducing the risk of wound infection. Equally, enthusiastic pre-operative prophylaxis commenced some days before prosthetic heart valve replacement has resulted in a higher rate of prosthetic endocarditis than in patients not receiving such treatment. Many outbreaks of surgical cross infection, due to such organisms as *Klebsiella* spp., have only been controlled following withdrawal of routine antibiotic prophylaxis.

However, there are certain areas in which prophylaxis is of value, for example:
1) Metronidazole in bowel and pelvic surgery (see section 16.4).
2) Staphylococcal prosthetic valve endocarditis where cloxacillin, used for 3 to 4 weeks, *commencing immediately prior to surgery,* has dramatically reduced the incidence of this complication.
3) Clostridal wound infection, where penicillin has virtually abolished this dangerous complication of hip surgery and lower limb amputation.
4) Burn sepsis, where simple topical agents such as silver nitrate 0.5% solution or silver sulphadiazine cream have done much to prevent *Ps. aeruginosa* infections.

Prophylaxis should be commenced just prior to surgery so that overgrowth of resistant variants does not occur, and should not be used in patients with an indwelling foreign body, for example, urinary catheter, which may allow the entry of a resistant organism.

24.2 Pyrexia Following Surgery

Many patients develop bacterial infections unrelated to their primary surgical problem, of which hypostatic pneumonia, urinary tract infection complicating catheterisation and infections of intravenous infusion sites are the most common. Pyrexia may also be due to non-infective causes such as deep vein thrombosis or myocardial infarction.

However, most patients developing pyrexia after surgery do so as a result of wound infection. Pyrexia early in convalescence, often within the immediate postoperative hours as in genitourinary surgery, associated with systemic upset or sudden collapse, is due to Gram-negative septicaemia and requires prompt treatment (see section 18).

Pyrexia which follows surgery after an interval of some days is due to wound infection or deep abscess formation, which may or may not be accompanied by bacteraemia. After bowel or gynaecological surgery, the infecting organisms are commonly anaerobes (see section 19) but after orthopaedic or neurosurgery Gram-positive or opportunist Gram-negative rods predominate. In all cases management is primarily directed to localisation and drainage of pus, antibiotic therapy occupying a secondary role in the control of attendant bacteraemia or tissue invasion, *if these are present*. Antibiotics are of no other value in deep seated abscesses except in staphylococcal infection complicating orthopaedic surgery or neurosurgery, where a combined approach of drainage and specific antistaphylococcal therapy is required.

25. Opportunistic Infection

The medical expression 'opportunistic infection' may be misleading for it is used in the sense of 'convenient access', as in the original Latin root, rather than the later 'appropriate' or 'favourable'.

Any of a great number of micro-organisms may gain access to the human body under one of a variety of predisposing circumstances. When the organism is derived from the patient's own natural flora the infection is termed endogenous, while exogenous opportunistic infection arises from the introduction of organisms into the compromised patient from his external environment.

25.1 Exogenous Opportunistic Infection

This occurs more frequently than endogenous infection, particularly in patients treated in the technologically advanced units of hospitals. The increasing use of surgical implants of various kinds has introduced special problems but the most commonly encountered exogenous infections are those associated with the use of intravenous cannulae and urinary catheters.

25.1.1 Intravenous Cannulae

Intravenous cannulae are a common source of local and invasive infection, which may be due to commensal organisms or to cross infection via medical or paramedical attendants. Bacterial contamination of intravenous fluids is uncommon but may result in Gram-negative septicaemia and death.

Prevention is dependent on:
1) An awareness of the risks
2) Scrupulous care in the placement and subsequent handling of the cannula site
3) Regular changing of the site to alternative veins at intervals which should not exceed 2 to 3 days
4) Avoidance of anastomoses in external tubing, which are potent sources of contamination
5) Extreme care when adding drugs to infusions.

Infusion sites require the same care and sterile precautions as are taken with surgical wounds and adequate skin preparation, preferably with iodine containing solutions, is of major importance. Topical prophylaxis with antibiotic sprays and creams should be avoided as their use may encourage *Candida* infection.

Local suppuration or cellulitis at the site of the cannula is most commonly due to staphylococci or streptococci, the latter commonly causing ascending lymphangitis. Septicaemia may follow such events but more commonly complicates indwelling transvenous cannulae in debilitated patients who are receiving antibiotics or parenteral feeding. In these circumstances opportunistic organisms such as *Pseudomonas* spp., members of the Klebsiella-Enterobacter-Serratia group, and Gram-negative cocci are frequently encountered. In patients receiving total parenteral nutrition (parenteral hyperalimentation) over 50 % of septicaemias are due to *Candida* spp.

In any patient with an indwelling venous cannula, unexplained pyrexia may indicate infection at this site and the cannula should be removed and sent *in its entirety*, together with blood for culture, for bacteriological investigation. Signs of septicaemia are an indication for immediate antibiotic therapy with a choice of drugs to cover the possibilities outlined above (for example cloxacillin and gentamicin) pending bacteriological advice. The management of *Candida* septicaemia requires expert assistance.

25.1.2 Urinary Catheters

The risk of inducing urinary tract infection by catheterisation has been assessed as 5 % following single catheterisation, 40 to 50 % after a 48 hour period of catheterisation and 100 % after 1 week. In obstetric or diabetic patients single

catheterisation carries a higher risk. Following bladder or prostatic surgery closed ir-
rigation has reduced the incidence of infection but the risk remains significant. In
patients with indwelling urinary catheters infection may be autogenous or may be
due to cross infection via medical attendants. In both cases infection ascends to the
bladder between the catheter and the urethral mucosa.

Antibiotic prophylaxis is of little use in genitourinary surgery, single catheterisation or cystoscopy, as the organisms which enter the bladder most often do so from
the perineal skin which may be 'sterilised' more effectively by local measures.

Once infection is established in catheterised patients antibiotics are contraindicated unless the infection is accompanied by systemic invasion. Cystitis associated
with catheters should not be treated with antibiotics as resistant superinfection is
likely to supervene and side effects may be produced unnecessarily. Bladder washouts
with chlorhexidine will reduce the viable count of bacteria and a high urine flow
should be encouraged. Systemic invasion and bacteraemia are discussed in section
25.3.

25.1.3 Infections of Prostheses

Surgical implantation of prosthetic devices may be complicated by infection with
opportunist pathogens introduced at operation. Infective endocarditis complicates
prosthetic heart valve replacement in 2 to 4% of cases. In two-thirds this is due to
staphylococci, commonly *Staph. albus*, but may also be due to Gram-negative bacilli
or to fungi such as *Candida* or *Aspergillus* spp. *Staph. albus* is also the most frequently encountered pathogen in infections of CSF shunts with Spitz-Holter and
other valves inserted to treat hydrocephalus. Prosthetic joint replacement may be
followed by immediate infection with Gram-positive cocci implanted at operation, or
by infection with either Gram-positive cocci or Gram-negative bacilli presenting
some months after surgery. The pathogenesis of these late infections is obscure.

Infection of a prosthesis is a disaster for the patient. The infection is unlikely to
be eradicated unless the prosthesis is removed, and therefore the patient will require a
further operation in circumstances where an increased risk of morbidity obtains.
Combined medical and surgical management is best left to teams experienced in the
treatment of such problems.

25.1.4 Infections Associated with Injections

Multiple intravenous injections may allow access of skin commensals to the cir-
culation. Local thrombophlebitis may be due to injected drugs, but may also be due to
such infection. In haemodialysis patients the access shunt may become infected,
usually with *Staph. aureus*, less commonly with *Staph. albus* or Gram-negative
bacilli. Endocarditis due to these organisms may rapidly supervene and this complication results in the death of 1 to 2% of patients on haemodialysis.

Local perivenous skin abscesses are a common accompaniment of intravenous drug abuse, and resultant bacteraemia may give rise to right sided endocarditis, which is a major complication of addiction. Mistaken injection of a peripheral artery may result in infective thrombosis and extensive gangrene. Infections associated with addiction are usually due to skin commensals and not to those organisms which contaminate 'street' heroin and 'unsuitable' diluents.

25.2 Endogenous Opportunistic Infection

This occurs when an organism, bacterial or viral, previously harboured in a physiological site gains entry to a pathological one; for example, on the entry into the bloodstream of enterobacteriaceae from the normal physiological habitat of the colon, with metastatic and systemic upsets of serious degree, very often seen in patients debilitated by disease of the colon itself, such as diverticular disease, Crohn's disease or ulcerative colitis. Similarly, should the pneumococcus pass from its normal physiological position in the upper posterior nasopharynx, either by droplet infection into the lungs or by passage through a skull defect to the meninges, serious morbidity, and sometimes mortality, ensues.

25.2.1 Predisposing Conditions: General

The healthy human fetus is sterile, but upon emerging from the womb the baby is rapidly colonised by micro-organisms, and the healthy baby acquires potential pathogens which live in symbiosis with it. For example, *Staphylococcus albus*, or even *Staphylococcus aureus*, colonise the skin, the pneumococcus resides in the upper posterior nasopharynx, and the large bowel is colonised by enterobacteriaceae in vast numbers. If these micro-organisms invade the body from the 'normal' sites to 'abnormal' sites, morbidity and mortality will invariably ensue (Gould, 1971). Thus, endogenous infections caused by these commensal bacteria can carry high mortality, especially in the preterm infant, the aged debilitated, the immunosuppressed, the traumatically shocked, or those subjected to massive surgical programmes. Endogenous infection is particularly common in diabetics and alcoholics, and since both diseases are very common, any deterioration in such a patient's physical state should not simply be blamed on the underlying disease process — a high degree of suspicion of endogenous infection should always be present in the clinician's mind. The ingestion of alcohol depresses the leucocytes in the peripheral blood *pari passu* with the amount ingested. Since alcoholics are particularly liable to head injuries, with the poor leucocyte defence resulting from alcoholic excess a coma may rapidly become complicated by the ingress of the pneumococcus, especially through the cribriform plate, leading to meningitis which carries a significant mortality despite the organism's high *in vitro* susceptibility to benzylpenicillin. The rapid appearance of gummy exudate around the base of the brain does not allow penicillin access to the pneumococcus in significant quantities. Thus, early diagnosis of pneumococcal meningitis, especially in the alcoholic, is fundamental to reducing mortality by the early institution of treatment.

25.2.2 Predisposing Conditions: Neutropenia

Neutropenia is frequently complicated by opportunistic infection. Decreasing neutrophil counts below $500/mm^3$ are associated with an exponential increase in infective episodes, and in some conditions, notably haematological malignancies producing neutropenia, the mortality of these infections exceeds 50%. Where tumours alter normal anatomy, such as the obstruction of a bronchus or of the urinary tract, local infection may result in a focus from which systemic spread may rapidly supervene.

Infections in neutropenics are usually endogenous, but exogenous infection may be acquired from the hospital environment via other patients, medical attendants or in seemingly inocuous vehicles such as hospital food, infusion fluids or paediatric feeds. Endogenous infections involve both aerobic and anaerobic Gram-negative bacilli from the bowel, and Gram-positive cocci from the skin and mucous membranes. Acquired hospital pathogens are almost exclusively Gram-negative bacilli such as *Klebsiella*, *Serratia*, *Acetinobacter* and *Pseudomonas* species. Fungi are occasionally involved.

Preventive measures are of paramount importance. The following measures are of *proven* value:

1) Reduction of skin contamination by chlorhexidine baths and creams

2) Reduction of the numbers of bacteria in the bowel by the use of non-absorbable antibiotic regimens, for example FRACON (framycetin, colomycin and nystatin in combination)

3) Use of sterile feeds, either as properly heated meals, sterilised tube feeds or elemental diets.

The use of isolation in the prevention of opportunistic infection does not seem to have the effectiveness originally attributed to it, and complete barrier systems such as the Trexler plastic isolator are probably not indicated. This does not mean that simple barrier precautions to prevent cross infection should be discarded.

Other methods of prophylaxis, such as the use of immuno-modulating agents (for example, levamisole and transfer factor), and prophylactic neutrophil transfusion are as yet unproven. However, the use of neutrophil transfusion may be life saving in established infection.

25.3 Bacteraemia

Gram-negative shock syndromes are second only to cardiogenic shock in incidence in modern medical practice (Murdoch et al., 1968). The transfer of antibiotic resistance between species of enterobacteriaceae is now well recognised and septicaemias resulting therefrom may be sensitive to only very few antibiotics, or even to none at all.

An analysis of approximately 300 patients with bacteraemia presenting in the 8-year period 1960 to 1967 at the Infectious Diseases Unit of the City Hospital, Edinburgh provides information about the frequency, causes and outcome of this type of infection.

25.3.1 Incidence

The overall incidence of bacteraemia was 15.5 per 1000 admissions. There was an increase from 3.4 per 1000 in 1960 to 12.9 per 1000 in 1967. In 1963, because of a local outbreak of paratyphoid fever, a peak incidence of 33.4 per 1000 admissions occurred. Excluding 1963, the highest rate was in 1965 with 55 cases or 23.7 per 1000 admissions. In all, 297 patients, 163 female and 134 male, were found to have bacteraemia. Gram-negative bacteraemia predominated in females (55:27) a ratio of 2:1. There were more females than males with salmonella bacteraemia (62:48), but slightly more males among the patients with Gram-positive coccal bacteraemia (52:43).

Ages ranged from 7 days to 88 years. 34 patients (11%) were older than 70 years. Among the patients with Gram-negative rod bacteraemia 54% were older than 50 years, 39% older than 60 years and only 7% younger than 3 years. In Gram-positive coccal bacteraemia patients, 39% were older than 50 years, 26% older than 60 years and 17% younger than 3 years. Only 16% of patients with salmonella bacteraemia were older than 50 years and 14% younger than 3 years. In bacteraemias due to meningococcus or *Haemophilus influenzae*, only children were involved, the oldest being 15 years.

25.3.2 Underlying Conditions

Urinary tract infection was the most common condition leading to Gram-negative bacteraemia, being present in 45 patients. A further 7 had cholangiohepatitis, 4 had nonspecific enteritis, 2 ulcerative colitis, 2 subphrenic abscesses, 2 diverticulitis, 2 pelvic abscesses and 1 had hepatic cirrhosis. One patient had just sustained a septic abortion and another had acute vaginitis. A variety of conditions were present in a further 16 patients, including malignant disease in 4 and other debilitating diseases in 12, while 3 patients were receiving corticosteroids.

In patients with Gram-positive coccal bacteraemia, respiratory infection was the most common underlying condition, being present in 39 patients. Skin sepsis occurred in 18 patients, all of whom had staphylococcal bacteraemia. Skeletal sepsis occurred in 12 patients, again due to the staphylococcus. 7 patients had endocarditis — streptococcal in 3, staphylococcal in 3 and pneumococcal in one. 5 patients had meningitis — pneumococcal in 4 and staphylococcal in one. 5 patients had non-specific gastro-enteritis and a further 5 had peritonitis. In 9 patients disorders reducing host defences were present — 5 had diabetes, 2 malignant disease and 1 each had myelomatosis and hypogammaglobulinaemia. 2 patients were receiving cortico-steroids.

The primary disease in all patients with salmonella bacteraemia was enteric fever.

In a miscellaneous group, a variety of primary conditions was present, including meningitis in 3 patients, brucellosis (3), subacute bacterial endocarditis (1), Weil's disease (1), canicola fever (1), pelvic peritonitis (1) and 1 patient was receiving cortico-steroids.

The probable portal of entry of the organisms responsible for bacteraemia was usually indicated by the primary disorder but it could not be determined accurately in 48 patients — 15 with Gram-negative bacteraemia, 24 with Gram-positive coccal bacteraemia and in 9 of the miscellaneous group.

25.3.3 Treatment

Gram-negative Bacteraemia
Antibacterial therapy was given to 72 patients: kanamycin to 33, cephaloridine to 23, chloramphenicol to 6, colistin to 3, lincomycin to 3, ampicillin to 2, benzylpenicillin to 2, cycloserine to 2, nitrofurantoin to 1 and erythromycin to 1. Single drug therapy was employed in most cases. 10 patients received no drugs. The standard adult dose for kanamycin was 250mg 6-hourly, for cephaloridine 500mg 6-hourly and for colistin 1.5 million units 8-hourly, all by the intramuscular route, for periods not exceeding 14 days. The standard doses were modified for age, body weight and state of renal function when indicated.

Gram-positive Bacteraemia
In this group 92 out of 95 patients were given antibiotics: benzylpenicillin to 28, lincomycin to 24, erythromycin to 19, cephaloridine to 18, methicillin to 8, kanamycin to 7, cloxacillin to 5 and chloramphenicol to 3. A few patients received more than 1 antibiotic consecutively. The dose of penicillin was dependent upon the organism and the primary disease. Pneumococcal bacteraemia arising in pneumonia was treated with 100,000 units 6-hourly intramuscularly for at least 4 days, followed by phenoxymethylpenicillin, 250mg 6-hourly orally, until full recovery. If pneumococcal meningitis was present, 500,000 units 4 to 6 hourly of penicillin were

given intramuscularly for at least 2 weeks. In subacute endocarditis due to *Strep-tococcus viridans* 1.5 to 4 million units were given intramuscularly daily with oral probenecid. Lincomycin was given in a dose of 500mg 6-hourly orally, often preceded by intramuscular and, occasionally, intravenous injections of 300 to 600mg 6 to 8 hourly. If osteomyelitis was present this antibiotic was continued for at least 6 weeks. The standard adult dose of erythromycin was 1 to 2g daily of the estolate for 14 days. Methicillin was given, 1g 4-hourly by intramuscular injection and cloxacillin 0.5g 4 to 6 hourly, usually orally, but initially by injection. Kanamycin and cephaloridine were used as in Gram-negative bacteraemia.

Salmonella Bacteraemia

Chloramphenicol and ampicillin were each used in 58 patients. The dose of chloramphenicol was 75mg/kg/24 hours up to a total of 2g daily for 14 days. Ampicillin was given in doses of 150mg/kg/24 hours up to 6g daily for 14 days.

Miscellaneous Bacteraemia

Each case was judged on its own merits and various antibiotics were used in standard dosage.

Treatment Other Than Antibacterials

Where a patient had been receiving corticosteroids prior to becoming bacteraemic, these drugs were continued. This arose in 5 patients. A further 13 who developed vasomotor collapse were given hydrocortisone in doses of 400mg daily. Vasopressors were used in only 7 patients and low molecular weight dextran in 6 patients with vasomotor collapse. Blood was transfused in 13 patients and other intravenous fluids were required in 33 dehydrated patients. Emergency surgery was necessary in 11 patients. Heparin was given to 1 patient with intravascular coagulation defect and, together with phenindione, to 2 patients with deep venous thrombosis.

25.3.4 Outcome of Treatment

Of the 297 patients, 47 died, giving an overall mortality of 15% — 22% for Gram-negative rod bacteraemia, 23% for Gram-positive bacteraemia, 3% for salmonella bacteraemia and 14% for the miscellaneous group. The interaction of the various factors influencing mortality such as age, sex, presence of vasomotor collapse, prior debilitating disease and the treatment given, makes evaluation of the efficacy of treatment almost impossible.

25.3.5 Interpretation of Results

This study shows an increase in all bacteraemic groups for the period 1960-67 and the rise would appear to be due to an increase in situations predisposing to bacteraemia. This confirms the findings in previous studies that the most important factor determining the outcome in patients with bacteraemia is the seriousness of the host condition (McCabe and Jackson, 1962a,b; Freid and Vosti, 1968). Prompt and appropriate antibacterial therapy significantly increases the chance of survival in patients with bacteraemia. In Gram-negative bacteraemia, experience showed that the prompt administration of either kanamycin or cephaloridine was beneficial. When pseudomonas bacteraemia was suspected colistin was used as the drug of choice; ampicillin and chloramphenicol were used in salmonella bacteraemia, while benzylpenicillin was primarily used for pneumococcal, streptococcal and penicillin sensitive staphylococcal bacteraemias. Lincomycin, cephaloridine, erythromycin, methicillin or cloxacillin were used when bacteraemia was due to penicillin resistant organisms. The mortality rates in this series compare favourably with other series, but it would appear that the most important factor is the early administration of appropriate bactericidal, parenteral antibiotics before the organism has been isolated and identified in the laboratory. Supportive therapeutic measures did not play a significant part in affecting the outcome.

25.4 Management of Opportunistic Infection

Knowledge of the portal of entry of the organism is of value in determining, on clinical grounds alone, the likely pathogen of opportunistic infections, especially those leading to bacteraemia. This allows an intelligent, inspired guess as to which antibacterial drug should be given as primary treatment, before laboratory confirmation is forthcoming (Murdoch, 1972).

These points of importance have been further highlighted, and the literature reviewed, by Brumfitt (1972). It should be added that opportunistic infections whether endogenous or exogenous, will remain with us although species of micro-organism involved, whether bacterial, viral, rickettsial, protozoal (or a mixture of these) will change. A high index of suspicion of opportunistic infection will depend first on the clinical state of the patient, then recognition in the milieu of conditions favourable to the emergence of potentially pathogenic micro-organisms.

26. The Management of Tuberculosis

This subject has recently been admirably reviewed by Seaton (1978). As he says, all forms of tuberculosis should be treated in the same way, preferably with a chest physician in charge with experience in the problems of the management of antituber-culosis chemotherapy. He further points out that this is true of tuberculosis present-ing to surgeons, as early diagnosis will often prevent unnecessary surgery. There seems little doubt that drugs alone will be successful in the management of almost all cases of tuberculosis, irrespective of the system involved, provided certain prin-ciples are adhered to. Initially adequate specimens should be sent to the laboratory so that *Mycobacterium tuberculosis* can be cultured, identified, and its pattern of drug resis-tance, if any, estimated. This will take 6 to 8 weeks; during this time treatment should be commenced with drugs to which the organism is likely to be sensitive. This primary regimen is continued for at least 8 weeks, or until the drug sensitivities are known. Thereafter 2 drugs are given. Such treatment reduces infectivity quickly by a rapid kill of the organisms and prevents resistance. Careful supervision, probably initially as an inpatient, but more importantly with outpatients, should ensure that the patient is taking the drugs; all the oral drugs should be taken on a fasting stomach. Obvious close contacts should be screened for evidence of tuberculosis.

Triple therapy with isoniazid, rifampicin and ethambutol is preferred for the first 8 to 12 weeks. In some countries, to reduce expense, streptomycin may be substituted for either rifampicin or ethambutol. Ethambutol has largely superseded PAS in prim-ary triple therapy. Occasionally, rifampicin may have to be withdrawn because of toxicity or cost, but then treatment time will increase from 9 to 18 months, and so the cost-efficacy is not really altered; also there is less chance of the patient pursuing treatment for 18 months than for 9 months. Various alternative regimens have been tried but these are less satisfactory, although they may have to be used in difficult cases, or where short term therapy is dictated by economics. Two such suitable com-binations are: streptomycin, isoniazid and rifampicin and streptomycin, isoniazid and pyrazinamide.

Seaton (1978) has outlined in detail the problems of treating tuberculosis, especially in the patient who is a vagrant, alcoholic, or both, or where drug resistance is suspected because the patient has had unsatisfactory antituberculosis drugs before, or has been in contact with a patient harbouring resistant organisms. The patient should always be fully informed of the type of treatment he has to take, why he has to take it at certain times of the day, and for how long. Combination tablets are prefera-ble to ensure that more than one drug is taken at a time. Urine testing at monthly visits is one method of checking that the drugs are being taken. The alcoholic should be removed from temptation by being admitted to hospital, especially if he is taking potentially hepatotoxic drugs. Nowadays, intrathecal treatment is not necessary in the management of meningitis; the indications for surgical procedures are now rare.

Corticosteroids produce a feeling of well-being in the toxic patient but they should not be used routinely except to suppress hypersensitivity reactions and the development of stricture formation in renal tuberculosis, or adhesions in meningitis. If these aspects of the general management of the tuberculous patient are strictly adhered to, the cure rate should approach 100%.

References

1. General

Garrod, L.P.; Lambert, H.P. and O'Grady, F.: in Antibiotic and Chemotherapy, 4th ed. (Churchill Livingstone, Edinburgh and London 1973).

Hawking, F. and Richmond, M.H.: Principles of chemotherapy; in *Passmore and Robson* A Companion to Medical Studies, Chapter 20 (Blackwell Scientific Publications, Oxford and Edinburgh 1970).

Kucers, A. and Bennett, N. McK.: The Use of Antibiotics 2nd Ed William Heinemann Medical Books Ltd, London 1975).

Manten, A.: in Meyler and Herxheimer Side Effects of Drugs, Vol. 7, Chapter 25, p.335-403 (Excerpta Medica, Amsterdam 1972).

2. The Sulphonamides

Ball, A.P. and Wallace, E.T.: A ten year study of the sensitivities of urinary pathogens in a pyelonephritis unit. Journal of International Medical Research *2* (Suppl. 1): 18-22 (1974).

Beveridge, J.; Harris, M.; Wise, G. and Stevens, L.: Long acting sulphonamides associated with Stevens-Johnson syndrome. Lancet *2*: 593 (1964).

Carrol, U.M.; Bryan, P.A. and Robinson, R.J.: Stevens-Johnson syndrome associated with long acting sulphonamides. Journal of the American Medical Association *195*: 691-693 (1966).

Holten, E.; Vaage, L.; Neess, C.; Midtvedt, T. and Jyssum, K.: Sulphonamide resistant meningococci after sulphonamide prophylaxis among naval recruits in Norway. Scandinavian Journal of Infectious Diseases *1*: 185-189 (1969).

Leading Article: Lung disease caused by drugs. British Medical Journal *3*: 729-730 (1969).

Leading Article: Meningococcal Infections. British Medical Journal *3*: 295-296 (1974a).

Leading Article: Sulphasalazine-induced lung disease. Lancet *2*: 504-505 (1974b).

Murdoch, J. McC.: Toxicity of the Sulphonamides. Practitioner *194*: 26-30 (1965).

Reeves, D.S.: Laboratory and clinical studies with sulfametopyrazine as a treatment for bacteriuria in pregnancy. Journal of Antimicrobial Chemotherapy *1*: 171-186 (1975).

3. The Natural Penicillins

Ashford, W.A.; Golash, R.G. and Hemming, V.G.: Penicillinase-producing Neisseria gonorrhoeae. Lancet *2*: 657-658 (1976).

Baldwin, D.S.; Levine, B.B.; McCluskey, R.T. and Gallo, G.R.: Renal failure and interstitial nephritis due to penicillin and methicillin. New England Journal of Medicine *279*: 1245-1252 (1968).

Barber, M. and Rozwadowska-Dowzenko, M.: Infection by penicillin-resistant staphylococci. Lancet *2*: 641-644 (1948).

Barber, M.: Coagulase-positive staphylococci resistant to penicillin. Journal of Pathology and Bacteriology *59*: 373-384 (1947).

Brunner, F.P. and Frick, P.G.: Hypokalaemia, metabolic alkalosis and hypernatraemia due to 'massive' sodium penicillin therapy. British Medical Journal *4*: 550-552 (1968).

Contoyiannis, P. and Adamopoulos, D.A.: Penicillin-resistant *Neisseria meningitidis*. Lancet *1*: 462 (1974).

Crofton, J.W.: Some principles in the chemotherapy of bacterial infections. British Medical Journal *2*: 137-141 (1969).

Ettinger, E. and Kaye, D.: Systemic manifestations after a skin test with penicilloyl-polylysine. New England Journal of Medicine *271:* 1105-1106 (1964).

Fishman, L.S. and Hewitt, W.L.: The Natural Penicillins. Medical Clinics of North America *54:* 1081-1099 (1970).

Fishman, R.A.: Active transport and the blood-brain barrier to penicillin and related organic acids. Transactions of the American Neurological Association *89:* 51-55 (1964).

Fishman, R.A.: Blood-brain and CSF barriers to penicillin and related organic acids. Archives of Neurology *15:* 113-124 (1966).

Garrod, L.P.; Lambert, H.P. and O'Grady, F.: Penicillins 1. Natural; in Antibiotic and Chemotherapy, 4th ed, p.53, 55 (Churchill Livingstone, Edinburgh and London 1973).

Gilbert, D.N.; Gourley, R.; d'Agostino, A.; Goodnight, S.H. and Worthen, H.: Interstitial nephritis due to methicillin, penicillin and ampicillin. Annals of Allergy *28:* 378-385 (1970).

Goslings, W.R.O.: Introductory remarks in Advances in Penicillin Allergy and Immunology, Proceedings of the Symposium, Rotterdam, p.8 (Beecham Research Laboratories, 1970).

Hamilton-Miller, J.T.: Inhibition of β-lactamase: a continuing story. Journal of Antimicrobial Chemotherapy *3:* 195-196 (1977).

Hansman, D.; Glasgow, H.; Sturt, J.; Devitt, L. and Douglas, R.: Increased resistance to penicillin of pneumococci isolated from man. New England Journal of Medicine *284:* 175-177 (1971).

Kunin, C.M.: Clinical significance of protein binding of the penicillins. Annals of the New York Academy of Sciences *145:* 282-289 (1967).

Leading Article: Penicillins and nephropathy. Lancet *2:* 447 (1974).

Leading Article: Penicillinase-producing gonococci. Lancet *2:* 725-726 (1976).

Leading Article: Immunological tolerance to treat penicillin allergy? Lancet *2:* 943 (1976).

Lerner, P.I.; Smith, H. and Weinstein, L.: Penicillin neurotoxicity. Annals of the New York Academy of Sciences *145:* 310-317 (1967).

Levine, B.B. and Zolov, D.M.: Prediction of penicillin allergy by immunological testing. Journal of Allergy *43:* 231-244 (1969).

Lynn, B.: The Semi-synthetic Penicillins; in Antibiotica et Chemotherapia, Vol. 13,.p.131 (S. Karger, Basle and New York 1965).

Morrison, A.W.: Phenethicillin and benzylpenicillin in acute otitis media. British Medical Journal *2:* 8-11 (1961).

Munro, A.C.: Immunology of macromolecular residues in penicillins; in Advances in Penicillin Allergy and Immunology, Proceedings of the Symposium in Rotterdam, p.67-77 (Beecham Research Laboratories 1970).

Orchard, R.T. and Rooker, G.: Penicillin-hypersensitivity-nephritis. Lancet *1:* 689 (1974).

Park, J.T. and Strominger, J.L.: Mode of action of penicillin: Biochemical basis for the mechanism of action of penicillin and for its selective toxicity. Science *125:* 99-101 (1957).

Petz, L.D. and Fudenberg, H.H.: Coombs-positive hemolytic anaemia caused by penicillin administration. New England Journal of Medicine *274:* 171-178 (1966).

Phillips, I.: β-lactamase-producing, penicillin-resistant gonococcus. Lancet *2:* 656-657 (1976).

Rolinson, G.N.: The significance of protein binding of penicillins; in *Brumfitt and Williams* Therapy with the New Penicillins, p.20 (Fellowship of Post Graduate Medicine, London 1964).

Shaltiel, S.; Mizrahi, R. and Sela, M.: On the immunological properties of penicillins. Proceedings of the Royal Society of London *179:* 411-432 (1971).

Smith, H.: in Antibiotics in Clinical Practice, p.208 (Pitman Medical, London 1972).

Spratt, B.G.: The action of mecillinam. Journal of Antimicrobial Chemotherapy *3* (Suppl. B): 13-19 (1977).

White, J.M.; Brown, D.L.; Hepner, G.W. and Worlledge, S.M.: Penicillin-induced haemolytic anaemia. British Medical Journal *3:* 26-29 (1968).

4. The Semi-synthetic Penicillins

Baldwin, D.S.; Levine, B.B.; McCluskey, R.T. and Gallo, G.R.: Renal failure and interstitial nephritis due to penicillin and methicillin. New England Journal of Medicine *279*: 1245-1252 (1968).

Bear, D.M.; Turck, M. and Petersdorf, R.G.: Ampicillin. Medical Clinics of North America *54*: 1145-1159 (1970).

Bond, J.M.; Lightbrown, J.W.; Barber, M. and Waterworth, P.M.: Four phenoxypenicillins. British Medical Journal *2*: 956-961 (1963).

Brauninger, G.E. and Remington, J.S.: Neuropathy associated with methicillin therapy. Journal of the American Medical Association *203*: 103-105 (1968).

Brogden, R.N. and Avery, G.S.: New Antibiotics: Epicillin, minocycline and spectinomycin. A summary of their antibacterial activity, pharmacokinetic properties and therapeutic efficacy. Drugs *3*: 314-330 (1972).

Brogden, R.N.; Speight, T.M. and Avery, G.S.: Amoxycillin: A review of its antibacterial and pharmacokinetic properties and therapeutic use. Drugs *9*: 88-140 (1975).

Cameron, S.J. and Richmond, J.: Ampicillin hypersensitivity in lymphatic leukaemia. Scottish Medical Journal *16*: 425-427 (1971).

Clayton, J.P.; Cole, M.; Elson, S.W. and Ferres, H.: BRL 8988 (talampicillin), a well-absorbed oral form of ampicillin. Antimicrobial Agents and Chemotherapy *5*: 670-671 (1974).

Clymo, A.B. and Harper, I.A.: Ampicillin-resistant *Haemophilus influenzae* meningitis. Lancet *1*: 453-454 (1974).

Collaborative Study Group: Prospective study of ampicillin rash. British Medical Journal *1*: 7-9 (1973).

Daehne, W.V.; Godtfredsen, W.O.; Roholt, K. and Tybring, L.: Pivampicillin, a new orally active ampicillin ester. Antimicrobial Agents and Chemotherapy 1970, p.431 (1971).

Dahnsjo, H.; Andersson, H.; Hallander, H.O. and Rudberg, R.D.: Tone audiometry control of children treated for meningitis with large intravenous doses of ampicillin. Acta Paediatrica Scandinavica *65*: 733-737 (1976).

Garrod, L.P.; Lambert, H.P. and O'Grady, F.: in Antibiotic and Chemotherapy, 4th ed, p.72 and 76 (Churchill Livingstone, Edinburgh and London 1973).

Gilbert, D.N. and Sanford, J.P.: Methicillin. Critical appraisal after a decade of experience. Medical Clinics of North America *54*: 1113-1125 (1970).

Hambleton, G. and Davies, Pamela A.: Diagnosis and management of bacterial meningitis. Drugs *8*: 15-53 (1974).

Heineman, H.S. and Israel, W.: Carbenicillin in the first nine months of unrestricted use. A chapter in the natural history of an antibiotic. Journal of Clinical Pharmacology *12*: 241-248 (1972).

Hewitt, W.L. and Winters, R.E.: The current status of parenteral carbenicillin. Journal of Infectious Diseases *127*: 120-129 (1973).

Kjellander, J.O. and Finland, M.: Studies of the penicillinase of *Staphylococcus albus*. Proceedings of the Society for Experimental Biology (N.Y.) *113*: 1031-1037 (1963).

Knudsen, E.T. and Harding, J.W.: A multicentre comparative trial of talampicillin and ampicillin in general practice. British Journal of Clinical Practice *29*: 255-266 (1975).

Lacey, R.: A new type of penicillin resistance of *Staphylococcus aureus?* Journal of Antimicrobial Chemotherapy *3*: 380-381 (1977).

Leading Article: An oral carbenicillin. British Medical Journal *3*: 555-556 (1973).

Leading Article: Haemophilus influenzae. Lancet *2*: 776-777 (1976).

Levitt, B.H.; Gottlieb, A.J.; Rosenberg, I.R. and Klein, J.J.: Bone marrow depression due to methicillin, a semisynthetic penicillin. Clinical Pharmacology and Therapeutics *5*: 301-306 (1964).

Marcy, S.M. and Klein, J.O.: The Isoxazolyl Penicillins: Oxacillin, Cloxacillin and Dicloxacillin. Medical Clinics of North America *54*: 1127-1143 (1970).

May, J.R. and Ingold, A.: Amoxicillin in the treatment of infections of the lower respiratory tract. Journal of Infectious Diseases *129* (Suppl. June): 189-193 (1974).

Neu, H.C.: Antimicrobial activity and human pharmacology of amoxycillin. Journal of Infectious Diseases *129* (Suppl): 123-131 (1974).

Parker, M.T. and Hewitt, J.H.: Methicillin resistance in *Staphylococcus aureus*. Lancet *1*: 800-804 (1970).

Pullen, H.; Wright, N. and Murdoch, J. McC.: Hypersensitivity reactions to antibacterial drugs in infectious mononucleosis. Lancet *2*: 1176-1178 (1967).

Rolinson, G.N.; Stevens, S.; Batchelor, F.R.; Wood, J.C. and Chain, E.B.: Bacteriological studies on a new penicillin BRL 1241. Lancet *2*: 564-567 (1960).

Schiffer, M.S.; MacLowry, J.; Schneerson, R.; Robbins, J.B.; McReynolds, J.W.; Thomas, W.J.; Bailey, D.W.; Clarke, E.J.; Mueller, E.J. and Escamilla, J.: Clinical, bacteriological and immunological characterisation of ampicillin-resistant *Haemophilus influenzae* type B. Lancet *2*: 257-259 (1974).

Sutherland, R. and Rolinson, G.N.: Characteristics of methicillin-resistant staphylococci. Journal of Bacteriology *87*: 887-899 (1964).

Sutherland, R.; Croydon, E.A.P. and Rolinson, G.N.: Amoxycillin: a new semi-synthetic penicillin. British Medical Journal *3*: 13-16 (1972).

Swarz, H. and Storari, F.E.: Indanyl carbenicillin. Excerpta Medica (1974).

The Medical Letter on Drugs and Therapeutics: Hetacillin *13*: 49-50 (Issue 324) (1971).

Turk, D.C.: Ampicillin-resistant *Haemophilus influenzae* meningitis. Lancet *1*: 453 (1974).

Wilcox, J.B.; Brogden, R.N. and Avery, G.S.: Pivampicillin: A preliminary report of its pharmacokinetic properties and therapeutic efficacy. Drugs *6*: 94-103 (1973).

5. Mecillinam and Pivmecillinam

Anderson, J.D.: Mecillinam resistance in clinical practice — a review. Journal of Antimicrobial Chemotherapy *3* (Suppl. B): 89-96 (1977).

Bresky, B.: Controlled randomized study comparing amoxycillin and pivmecillinam in adult out-patients presenting with symptoms of acute urinary tract infection. Journal of Antimicrobial Chemotherapy *3* (Suppl. B): 121-127 (1977).

Clarke, P.D.; Geddes, A.M.; McGhie, D. and Wall, J.C.: Mecillinam: a new antibiotic for enteric fever. British Medical Journal *2*: 14-15 (1976).

Geddes, A.M. and Clarke, P.D.: The treatment of enteric fever with mecillinam. Journal of Antimicrobial Chemotherapy *3* (Suppl. B): 101-102 (1977).

Guttmann, D.: A comparison of pivmecillinam and co-trimoxazole in the treatment of simple cystitis in general practice. Journal of Antimicrobial Chemotherapy *3* (Suppl. B): 137-140 (1977).

Ishigami, J.: Clinical evaluation of pivmecillinam in acute simple cystitis: a comparative study with amoxycillin by a randomized double-blind technique. Journal of Antimicrobial Chemotherapy *3* (Suppl. B): 129-135 (1977).

Jonsson, M.: Pivmecillinam in the treatment of *Salmonella* carriers. Journal of Antimicrobial Chemotherapy *3* (Suppl. B): 103-107 (1977).

Leading Article: Mecillinam. Lancet *2*: 503-505 (1976).

Lund, F. and Tybring, L.: 6β-amidinopenicillanic acids — a new group of antibiotics. Nature New Biology *236*: 135-137 (1972).

Mecillinam. Journal of Antimicrobial Chemotherapy *3* (Suppl. B): 1-160 (1977).

Mitchard, M.; Andrews, J.; Kendall, M.J. and Wise, R.: Mecillinam serum levels following intravenous injection: a comparison with pivmecillinam. Journal of Antimicrobial Chemotherapy *3* (Suppl. B): 83-88 (1977).

Neu, H.C.: Mecillinam — an amidino penicillin which acts synergistically with other β-lactam compounds. Journal of Antimicrobial Chemotherapy *3* (Suppl. B): 43-52 (1977).

Pines, A.; Nandi, A.R.; Raafat, H. and Rahman, M.: Pivmecillinam and amoxycillin as combined treat-

ment in purulent exacerbation of chronic bronchitis. Journal of Antimicrobial Chemotherapy *3*
    (Suppl. B): 141-148 (1977).

Roholt, K.: Pharmacokinetic studies with mecillinam and pivmecillinam. Journal of Antimicrobial
    Chemotherapy *3* (Suppl. B): 71-81 (1977).

Spratt, B.G.: The mechanism of action of mecillinam. Journal of Antimicrobial Chemotherapy *3* (Suppl.
    B): 13-19 (1977).

Verrier Jones, E.R. and Asscher, A.W.: Treatment of recurrent bacteriuria with pivmecillinam (FL1039).
    Journal of Antimicrobial Chemotherapy 1: 193-196 (1975).

Williams, J.D.; Andrews, J.; Mitchard, M. and Kendall, M.J.: Bacteriology and pharmacokinetics of the
    new amidino penicillin — mecillinam. Journal of Antimicrobial Chemotherapy *2:* 61-69 (1976).

Wise, R.; Pippard, M. and Reeves, D.S.: A laboratory and clinical investigation of u.   ·nd its
    ester pivmecillinam in the treatment of urinary tract infection. Journal of Antimicrc   mo-
    therapy *3* (Suppl. B): 113-120 (1977).

6. *Co-trimoxazole (trimethoprim-sulphamethoxazole*

Avery, G.S. (ed.): Trimethoprim-sulphamethoxazole. Drugs *1:* 8-53 (

Ball, A.P. and Wallace, E.T.: A ten year survey of the sensitivi.   . ·   , pathogens in a
    pyelonephritis unit. Journal of International Medical Research *2* (Suppl. 1): 18-22 (1974).

Bateson, M.C.; Hayes, J.P.L.A. and Pendharkar, P.: Co-trimoxazole and folate metabolism. Lancet *2:*
    339-340 (1976).

Bengtsson, E.; Svanbom, M. and Tunevall, G.: Trimethoprim-sulphamethoxazole. Treatment in staphy-
    lococcal endocarditis and Gram-negative septicaemia. Scandinavian Journal of Infectious Diseases
    16: 177-182 (1974).

Brumfitt, W. and Pursell, R.: Double blind trial to compare ampicillin, cephalexin, co-trimoxazole and tri-
    methoprim in treatment of urinary tract infection. British Medical Journal *2:* 673-676 (1972).

Burchall, J.J.: Mechanism of action of trimethoprim-sulphamethoxazole: I. Journal of Infectious Diseases
    128 (Suppl. Nov): 437-441 (1973).

Bushby, S.R.M.: Trimethoprim-sulphamethoxazole. *In vitro* microbiological aspects. Journal of Infectious
    Diseases *128* (Suppl. Nov): 442-462 (1973).

Cattell, W.R.; Chamberlain, D.A.; Fry, I.K.; McSherry, M.A.; Broughton, C. and O'Grady, F.: Long-
    term control of bacteriuria with trimethoprim-sulphonamide. British Medical Journal *1:* 377-379
    (1971).

Chanarin, I. and England, J.M.: Toxicity of trimethoprim-sulphamethoxazole in patients with
    megaloblastic haemopoiesis. British Medical Journal *1:* 651-653 (1972).

Daikos, G.K.; Papapolyzos, N.; Marketos, N.; Mochlas, S.; Kastanakis, S. and Papasteriadis, E.: Tri-
    methoprim-sulphamethoxazole in brucellosis. Journal of Infectious Diseases *128:* (Suppl. Nov):
    731-733 (1973).

Darrell, J.H.; Garrod, L.P. and Waterworth, P.M.: Trimethoprim: Laboratory and clinical studies. Jour-
    nal of Clinical Pathology *21:* 202-209 (1968).

Everett, E.D. and Kishimoto, R.A.: *In vitro* sensitivity of *Pseudomonas pseudomallei* to trimethoprim and
    sulphamethoxazole. Journal of Infectious Diseases *128* (Suppl. Nov): 539-542 (1973).

Feldman, H.A.: Effects of trimethoprim and sulphisoxazole alone and in combination on murine tox-
    oplasmosis. Journal of Infectious Diseases *128* (Suppl. Nov): 774-776 (1973).

Fleming, M.P.; Datta, N. and Gruneberg, R.N.: Trimethoprim resistance determined by R factors. British
    Medical Journal *1:* 726-728 (1972).

Geddes, A.M.; Fothergill, R.; Goodall, J.A.D. and Dorken, P.R.: Evaluation of trimethoprim-
    sulphamethoxazole in treatment of salmonella infections. British Medical Journal *3:* 451-454
    (1971).

Gilman, R.H.; Terminel, M.; Levine, M.L.; Hernandez-Mendoza, P.; Calderone, E.; Vasquez, V.; Martinez, E.; Snyder, M.J. and Hornick, R.B.: Comparison of trimethoprim-sulfamethoxazole and amoxycillin in therapy of chloramphenicol-resistant and chloramphenicol-sensitive typhoid fever. Journal of Infectious Diseases *132:* 630-636 (1975).

Gray, J.; McGhie, D. and Ball, A.P.: Data to be published (1977).

Gruneberg, R.N. and Kolbe, R.: Trimethoprim in the treatment of urinary infections in hospital. British Medical Journal *1:* 545-547 (1969).

Hall, C.L.: Cotrimoxazole and azathioprine: A safe combination. British Medical Journal *4:* 15-16 (1974).

Hanson, G.C. and Woods, R.L.: Intravenous trimethoprim/sulphadimidine in the treatment of Bacteroides septicaemia. Postgraduate Medical Journal *51:* 105-106 (1975).

Herbert, V.: Metabolism of folic acid in man. Journal of Infectious Diseases *128* (Suppl. Nov): 601-606 (1973).

Hitchings, G.H.: Mechanism of action of trimethoprim-sulphamethoxazole: II. Journal of Infectious Diseases *128* (Suppl. Nov): 433-435 (1973).

Hughes, D.T.D.: Use of combinations of trimethoprim and sulphamethoxazole in the treatment of chest infections. Journal of Infectious Diseases *128* (Suppl. Nov): 701-705 (1973).

Hughes, W.T.; Feldman, S. and Sanyal, S.K.: Treatment of pneumocystis carinii pneumonitis with trimethoprim-sulfamethoxazole. Canadian Medical Association Journal *112* (Suppl. June): 47S-50S (1975).

Hulme, B. and Reeves, D.S.: Leucopaenia associated with trimethoprim-sulphamethoxazole after renal transplantation. British Medical Journal *3:* 610-612 (1971).

Kahn, S.B.; Fein, S.A. and Brodsky, I.: Effects of trimethoprim on folate metabolism in man. Clinical Pharmacology and Therapeutics *9:* 550-560 (1968).

Kalowski, S.; Nanra, R.S.; Mathew, T.H. and Kincaid-Smith, P.: Deterioration in renal function in association with co-trimoxazole therapy. Lancet *1:* 394-397 (1973).

Kamat, S.A.: Evaluation of the therapeutic efficacy of trimethoprim-sulphamethoxazole and chloramphenicol in enteric fever. British Medical Journal *3:* 320-322 (1970).

Kaplan, S.A.; Weinfeld, R.E.; Abazzo, C.W.; McFaden, K.; Jack, M.L. and Weissman, L.: Pharmacokinetic profile of trimethoprim-sulphamethoxazole in man. Journal of Infectious Diseases *128* (Suppl. Nov): 547-555 (1973).

Kirwan, W.O.: Cerebrospinal fluid cotrimoxazole levels. Journal of the Irish Medical Association *67:* 76-77 (1974).

Lawrence, A.; Phillips, I. and Nicol, C.: Various regimens of trimethoprim-sulphamethoxazole in the treatment of gonorrhoea. Journal of Infectious Diseases *128* (Suppl. Nov): 673-678 (1973).

May, J.R. and Davies, J.: Resistance of *H. influenzae* to trimethoprim. British Medical Journal *3:* 376-377 (1972).

Meares, E.M.: Observations on activity of trimethoprim-sulphamethoxazole on the prostate. Journal of Infectious Diseases *128* (Suppl. Nov): 679-685 (1973).

Morzaria, R.N.; Walton, I.G. and Pickering, D.: Neonatal meningitis treated with trimethoprim and sulphamethoxazole. British Medical Journal *2:* 511 (1969).

Mossner, G.: Clinical results with the combined preparation sulphamethoxazole + trimethoprim. Proceedings of the 6th International Congress of Chemotherapy, Tokyo. *A11-2:* 250, abstract (1969).

Phillips, I. and Warren, C.: Susceptibility of bacteroides fragilis to trimethoprim and sulphamethoxazole. Lancet *1:* 827-828 (1974).

Pichler, H.; Knothe, H.; Spitzy, K.H. and Veilkind, G.: Treatment of chronic carriers of *Salmonella typhi* and *Salmonella paratyphi* B with trimethoprim-sulfamethoxazole. Journal of Infectious Diseases *128* (Suppl. Nov): 743-744 (1973).

Reeves, D.S.; Faiers, M.C.; Pursell, R.E. and Brumfitt, W.: Trimethoprim-sulphamethoxazole: Comparative study in urinary infections in hospital. British Medical Journal *1:* 541-544 (1969).

Rieder, J.: Excretion of sulphamethoxazole and trimethoprim into human bile. Journal of Infectious Diseases *128* (Suppl. Nov): 574-575 (1973).

Ruskin, J. and Remington, J.S.: Toxoplasmosis in the compromised host. Annals of Internal Medicine *84:* 193-199 (1976).

Sabel, K.-G. and Brandberg, A.: Treatment of meningitis and septicemia in infancy with a sulphamethoxazole/trimethoprim combination. Acta Paediatrica Scandinavica *64:* 25-32 (1975).

Schofield, C.B.S.; Masterton, G.; Moffat, M. and McGill, M.I.: Gonorrhoea in women. Treatment with sulphamethoxazole and trimethoprim. Journal of Infectious Diseases *124:* 533-538 (1971).

Schwartz, D.E. and Ziegler, W.H.: Assay and pharmacokinetics of trimethoprim in man and animals. Postgraduate Medical Journal *45* (Suppl. May): 32-37 (1969).

Scragg, J.N. and Rubidge, C.J.: Trimethoprim and sulphamethoxazole in typhoid fever in children. British Medical Journal *3:* 738-741 (1971).

Seligman, S.T.; Madhaven, T. and Alcid, D.: Trimethoprim-sulphamethoxazole in the treatment of bacterial endocarditis. Journal of Infectious Diseases *128* (Suppl. Nov): 754-761 (1973).

Sharpstone, P.: The renal handling of trimethoprim and sulphamethoxazole in man. Postgraduate Medical Journal *45* (Suppl. May): 32-37 (1969).

Smellie, J.M.; Gruneberg, R.N.; Leakey, A. and Atkin, W.S.: Long term low dosage co-trimoxazole in the management of urinary tract infection in children. Journal of Antimicrobial Chemotherapy *2:* 287-291 (1976).

Tasker, P.R.W.; McGregor, G.A.; De Wardener, H.E.; Thomas, R.D. and Jones, N.F.: Use of co-trimoxazole in renal failure. Lancet *1:* 1216-1218 (1975).

Then, R. and Angehrn, P.: Nature of the bactericidal action of sulphonamides and trimethoprim: Alone and in combination. Journal of Infectious Diseases *128* (Suppl. Nov): 498-501 (1973).

Udall, V.: Toxicology of sulphonamide trimethoprim combinations. Postgraduate Medical Journal *45* (Suppl. May): 42-45 (1969).

Welling, P.G.; Craig, W.A.; Amidon, G.L. and Kunin, C.M.: Pharmacokinetics of trimethoprim and sulphamethoxazole in normal subjects and in patients with renal failure. Journal of Infectious Diseases *128* (Suppl. Nov): 556-566 (1973).

Whitman, E.N.: Effects in man of prolonged administration of trimethoprim and sulfisoxazole. Postgraduate Medical Journal *45* (Suppl. May): 46-51 (1969).

Wilfert, C.M.: Trimethoprim-sulphamethoxazole in children. Pharmacokinetics and Clinical Studies. Journal of Infectious Diseases *128* (Suppl. Nov): 613-617 (1973).

Williams, J.D. and Andrews, J.: Sensitivity of *H. influenzae* to antibiotics. British Medical Journal *1:* 134-137 (1974).

7. Chloramphenicol

Cherubin, C.E.; Neu, H.C.; Rahal, J.J. and Sabath, L.D.: Emergence of resistance to chloramphenicol in Salmonella. Journal of Infectious Diseases *135:* 807-812 (1977).

Kucers, A.: Chloramphenicol; in The Use of Antibiotics, p.164-185 (William Heinemann Medical Books, London 1972).

Lampe, R.M.; Mansuwan, P. and Duangmani, C.: Chloramphenicol-resistant typhoid. Lancet *1:* 623-624 (1974).

Murdoch, J. McC.: Antibiotics and chemotherapy; in *Alstead and Girdwood* Textbook of Medical Treatment, 13th ed, p.56 (Churchill Livingstone, Edinburgh and London 1974).

8. Tetracyclines

Finland, M.: Twenty-fifth anniversary of the discovery of Aureomycin: The place of the tetracyclines in antimicrobial therapy. Clinical Pharmacology and Therapeutics *15:* 3-8 (1974).

Garrod, L.P.; Lambert, H.P. and O'Grady, R.: Tetracyclines; in Antibiotic and Chemotherapy, 4th ed, p.149-166 (Churchill Livingstone, Edinburgh and London 1973).

Kucers, A.: Tetracyclines; in The Use of Antibiotics, p.271-306 (William Heinemann Medical Books, London 1972).

Minuth, J.N.; Holmes, T.M. and Musher, D.M.: Activity of tetracycline, doxycycline, and minocycline against methicillin-susceptible and -resistant staphylococci. Antimicrobial Agents and Chemotherapy 6: 411 (1974).

Murdoch, J. McC.: The tetracyclines, in Alstead and Girdwood Textbook of Medical Treatment, 13th ed, p.52-55 (Churchill Livingstone, Edinburgh and London 1974).

9. The Macrolides

Bell, S.M.: A comparison of absorption after oral administration of erythromycin estolate and erythromycin stearate. Medical Journal of Australia 2: 1280-1283 (1971).

Garrod, L.P.: The erythromycin group of antibiotics. British Medical Journal 2: 57-63 (1957).

Garrod, L.P.; Lambert, H.P. and O'Grady, F.: Macrolides; in Antibiotic and Chemotherapy, 4th ed, p.170 (Churchill Livingstone, Edinburgh and London 1973).

Kucers, A.: Spiramycin, oleandomycin and kitasamycin; in The Use of Antibiotics, p.223 (William Heinemann Medical Books, London 1972).

Lacey, R.W.: A new look at erythromycin. Postgraduate Medical Journal 53: 195-200 (1977).

Lake, B. and Bell, S.M.: Variations in absorption of erythromycin. Medical Journal of Australia 1: 449-451 (1969).

Oleinick, N.L. and Corcoran, J.W.: Two types of binding of erythromycin to ribosomes from antibiotic-sensitive and -resistant Bacillus subtilis 168. Journal of Biological Chemistry 244: 727-735 (1969).

Scottish Medical Journal: Erythromycin Symposium Issue 22: 5 (1977).

Wiegand, R.G. and Chun, A.H.C.: Serum protein binding of erythromycin and erythromycin 2-propionate ester. Journal of Pharmaceutical Sciences 61: 425-428 (1972).

10. Lincomycin and Clindamycin

Cohen, L.E.; McNeill, C.J. and Wells, R.F.: Clindamycin associated colitis. Journal of the American Medical Association 223: 1379-1380 (1973).

Garrod, L.P.; Lambert, H.P. and O'Grady, F.: Lincomycin; in Antibiotic and Chemotherapy, 4th ed, p.208 and 212 (Churchill Livingstone, Edinburgh and London 1973).

Geddes, A.M.; Sleet, R.A. and Murdoch, J. McC.: Lincomycin. Hydrochloride: Clinical and laboratory studies. British Medical Journal 2: 660-664 (1964).

Geddes, A.M.; Dwyer, N. St. J.; Ball, A.P. and Amos, R.S.: Clindamycin in bone and joint infections. Journal of Antimicrobial Chemotherapy 3: 501-507 (1977).

Kaplan, K. and Weinstein, L.: Lincomycin. Pediatric Clinics of North America 15: 131-139 (1968).

McGehee, R.F.; Smith, C.B.; Wilcox, C. and Finland, M.: Comparative studies of antibacterial activity in vitro and absorption and excretion of lincomycin and clinimycin. American Journal of Medical Sciences 256: 279-292 (1968).

Novak, E.; Vitti, T.G.; Panzer, J.D.; Schlagel, C. and Hearron, M.S.: Antibiotic tolerance and serum levels after intravenous administration of multiple large doses of lincomycin. Clinical Pharmacology and Therapeutics 12: 793-797 (1971).

Phillips, I.; Fernandes, R. and Warren, Christine: In vitro comparison of erythromycin, lincomycin and clindamycin. British Medical Journal 2: 89 (1970).

Pittman, F.E.; Pittman, J.C. and Humphrey, C.D.: Lincomycin and pseudomembranous colitis. Lancet 1: 451-452 (1974).

Sanders, E.: Lincomycin: Fact, fantasy and future. Medical Clinics of North America *54:* 1295-1303 (1970).

Scott, A.J.; Nicholson, G.I. and Kerr, A.R.: Lincomycin as a cause of pseudomembranous colitis. Lancet *2:* 1232-1234 (1973).

Wagner, J.G.; Novak, E.; Patel, N.C.; Chidester, C.G. and Lummis, W.L.: Absorption, excretion and half-life of clinimycin in normal adult males. American Journal of Medical Sciences *256:* 25-37 (1968).

11. Fusidic Acid (Sodium Fusidate)

Garrod, L.P.; Lambert, H.P. and O'Grady, F.: Various Antibacterial Antibiotics — Fusidic Acid; in Antibiotic and Chemotherapy, 4th ed, p.201 and 204. (Churchill Livingstone, Edinburgh and London 1973).

Godtfredsen, W.; Roholt, K. and Tybring, L.: Fucidin: a new orally active antibiotic. Lancet *1:* 928 (1962).

Godtfredsen, W.O. and Vangedal, S.: On the metabolism of fusidic acid in man. Acta Chemica Scandinavica *20:* 1599-1607 (1966).

Harvey, C.L.; Knight, S.G. and Sih, C.J.: On the mode of action of fusidic acid. Biochemistry *5:* 3320-3327 (1966).

Hoeprich, P.D.; Benner, E.J. and Kayser, F.H.: Susceptibility of methicillin-resistant *Staphylococcus aureus* to 12 antimicrobial agents in Antimicrobial Agents and Chemotherapy, p.104 (1969).

Jensen, K. and Lassen, H.C.A.: Combined treatment with antibacterial chemotherapeutical agents in staphylococcal infections. Quarterly Journal of Medicine *38:* 91-106 (1969).

Kucers, A.: Fusidate sodium (Fucidin); in The Use of Antibiotics, p.188 (W. Heinemann Medical Books, London 1972).

Liddy, N.: Intravenous fusidic acid in the newborn. Lancet *1:* 621 (1973).

Lowbury, E.J.L.; Cason, J.S.; Jackson, D. MacG. and Miller, R.W.S.: Fucidin for staphylococcal infections of burns. Lancet *2:* 478-480 (1962).

Murdoch, J. McC.: Antibiotics and chemotherapy; in *Alstead and Girdwood* Textbook of Medical Treatment, 13th ed, p.44-68 (Churchill Livingstone, Edinburgh and London 1974).

O'Garra, J.A.: Methicillin-resistant staphylococci. Lancet *2:* 1037-1038 (1968).

O'Grady, F. and Greenwood, D.: Interactions between fusidic acid and penicillins. Journal of Medical Microbiology *6:* 441-450 (1973).

Wynn, V.: Metabolic effects of the steroid antibiotic fusidic acid. British Medical Journal *1:* 1400-1404 (1965).

12. Urinary Antiseptics

Adam, W.R. and Dawborn, J.K.: Plasma levels and urinary excretion of nalidixic acid in patients with renal failure. Australian and New Zealand Journal of Medicine *2:* 126-131 (1971).

Back, O.; Lundgren, R. and Wiman, L-G.: Nitrofurantoin-induced pulmonary fibrosis and lupus syndrome. Lancet *2:* 930 (1974).

Boreus, L.O. and Sundstrom, B.: Intracranial hypertension in a child during treatment with nalidixic acid. British Medical Journal *2:* 744-745 (1967).

Burman, L.G.: Apparent absence of transferable resistance to nalidixic acid in pathogenic Gram-negative bacteria. Journal of Antimicrobial Chemotherapy *3:* 509-516 (1977).

Finegold, S.M. and Ziment, I.: Sulfonamides, nitrofurans and nalidixic acid. Pediatric Clinics of North America *15:* 95-105 (1968).

Garrod, L.P.; Lambert, H.P. and O'Grady, F.: Nalidixic acid; in Antibiotic and Chemotherapy, 4th ed., p.38-41 (Churchill Livingstone, Edinburgh and London 1973).

Goff, J.B.; Schlegel, J.U. and O'Dell, R.M.: Urinary excretion of nalidixic acid, sulfamethiazole and nitrofurantoin in patients with reduced renal function. Journal of Urology 99: 371-375 (1968).

Kucers, A.: Nitrofurantoin; in The Use of Antibiotics, p.359-367. (William Heinemann Medical Books, London 1972).

Leading Article: Pulmonary sensitivity to nitrofurantoin. British Medical Journal 4: 704 (1969).

Loughridge, L.W: Peripheral neuropathy due to nitrofurantoin. Lancet 2: 1133-1135 (1962).

Lowentritt, L.L. and Schlegel, J.U.: Treatment of bacteriuria in patients with impaired renal function. Journal of Urology 102: 473-478 (1969).

Rosenow, E.C.; De Remee, R.A. and Dines, D.E.: Chronic nitrofurantoin pulmonary reaction. Report of five cases. New England Journal of Medicine 279: 1258-1262 (1968).

Sellers, E.M. and Koch-Weser, J.: Displacement of warfarin from human albumin by diazoxide and ethacrynic, mefenamic and nalidixic acids. Clinical Pharmacology and Therapeutics 11: 524 (1970).

Stamey, T.A.; Nemoy, N.J. and Higgins, M.: The clinical use of nalidixic acid. A review and some observations. Investigative Urology 6: 582-592 (1969).

Toole, J.F.; Gergen, J.A.; Hayes, D.M. and Felts, J.H.: Neural effects of nitrofurantoin. Archives of Neurology 18: 680-687 (1968).

Wren, B.G.: Sub-clinical renal infection in pregnancy: Pathogenesis, the organisms and the drugs of choice in its treatment. Medical Journal of Australia 2: 895-898 (1969).

Zinsser, H.H.: Nalidixic acid in acute and chronic urinary tract infection. Medical Clinics of North America 54: 1347-1350 (1970).

13. Cephalosporins

Ball, A.P. and Geddes, A.M.: In Advances in Infection. (Churchill Livingstone, Edinburgh and London 1978). In press.

Butler, M.: Clinical trial: Cephradine in the treatment of urinary tract infection. Journal of the Irish Medical Association 66 (Suppl. March 24): 13-15 (1973).

Eykyn, S.: Use and control of cephalosporins. Journal of Clinical Pathology 24: 419-429 (1971).

James, D.G. and Walker, A.: The cephalosporins. British Journal of Hospital Medicine 6: 795-804 (1971).

Kosmidis, J.; Hamilton-Miller, J.M.T.; Gilchrist, J.N.G.; Kerry, D.W. and Brumfitt, W.: Cefoxitin, a new semisynthetic cephamycin. An in vitro and in vivo comparison with cephalothin. British Medical Journal 4: 653-655 (1973).

Leading Article: Cephalosporins, present and future. Lancet 2: 364-365 (1973).

McLean, P.: Cephradine in the treatment of urinary tract infections. Journal of the Irish Medical Association 66 (Suppl. March 24): 16-17 (1973).

Martin, R.R.: Clinical experience with oral cephradine. Journal of the Irish Medical Association 66 (Suppl. March 24): 25-28 (1973).

Mogagab. W.J.: Use of cephradine in respiratory tract infections. Journal of the Irish Medical Association 66 (Suppl. March 24): 18-24 (1973).

Murdoch, J. McC.: Cephaloridine. The Practitioner 195: 109-113 (1965).

Neiss, E.S.: Cephradine — A summary of preclinical studies and clinical pharmacology. Journal of the Irish Medical Association 66 (Suppl. March 24): 1-12 (1973).

Quinn, E.L.; Freimer, E.H.; Cox, F.; Fisher, E.J. and Madhavan, T.: Clinical experience with cefazolin. Scientific Exhibit, Fifty-fourth Annual Session of the American College of Physicians, Chicago, Illinois, April 9-13 (1973).

Wise, R.: A guide to the cephalosporin antibiotics. British Journal of Hospital Medicine 11: 583-589 (1974).

14. Peptide Antibiotics (Polymyxins)

Garrod, L.P.; Lambert, H.P. and O'Grady, F.: Peptides; in Antibiotic and Chemotherapy, 4th ed, p.179 (Churchill Livingstone, Edinburgh and London 1973).

Goodwin, N.J.: Colistin and sodium colistimethate. Medical Clinics of North America 54: 1267-1276 (1970).

Hoeprich, P.R.: The polymyxins. Medical Clinics of North America 54: 1257-1265 (1970).

Jawetz, E.: Polymyxins, colistin, bacitracin, ristocetin and vancomycin. Pediatric Clinics of North America 15: 85-95 (1968).

Marsden, H.B. and Hyde, W.A.: Colistin methane sulphonate in childhood infections. Lancet 2: 740-742 (1962).

Naiman, J.G. and Martin, J.D.: Some aspects of neuromuscular blockade with polymyxin B. Journal of Surgical Research 7: 199-206 (1967).

Perkins, R.L.: Apnea with intramuscular colistin therapy. Journal of the American Medical Association 190: 421-424 (1964).

Prevoznik, S.J.: Truncal ataxia as a complication of colistin therapy: Its relation to spinal anaesthesia. Anaesthesia and Analgesia 46: 46-48 (1967).

Smith, H.: Miscellaneous antibiotics; in Antibiotics in Clinical Practice, p.102 (Pitman Medical, Bath 1972).

Wolinsky, E. and Hines, J.D.: Neurotoxic and nephrotoxic effects of colistin in patients with renal disease. New Zealand Journal of Medicine 266: 759-762 (1962).

15. Aminoglycosides

Association for the Study of Infectious Disease: Effect of neomycin in non-invasive salmonella infections of the gastro-intestinal tract. Lancet 2: 1159-1161 (1970).

Barber, M. and Waterworth, P.M.: Activity of gentamicin against Pseudomonas and hospital staphylococci. British Medical Journal 1: 203-204 (1966).

Barza, M.; Brown, R.B.; Shen, D.; Gibaldi, M. and Weinstein, L.: Predictability of blood levels of gentamicin in man. Journal of Infectious Diseases 132: 165-174 (1975).

Bendush, C.L. and Weber, R.: Tobramycin sulfate: a summary of worldwide experience from clinical trials. Journal of Infectious Diseases 134 (Suppl.): S219-234 (1976).

Berk, D.P.: Deafness complicating antibiotic therapy of hepatic encephalopathy. Annals of Internal Medicine 73: 393-396 (1970).

Bint, A.J.: Gentamicin resistant Staphylococcus aureus. Journal of Antimicrobial Chemotherapy 2: 225 (1976).

Black, H.R. and Griffiths, R.S.: Preliminary studies with nebramycin factor 6, in Antimicrobial Agents and Chemotherapy, p.314-321 (1970).

Blair, D.C.; Fekety, F.R.; Bruce, B.; Silva, J. and Archer, G.: Therapy of Pseudomonas aeruginosa infections with tobramycin. Antimicrobial Agents and Chemotherapy 8: 22-29 (1975).

Breen, K.J.; Bryant, R.E.; Levinson, J.D. and Schenker, S.: Neomycin absorption in man. Annals of Internal Medicine 70: 211-218 (1972).

Britt, M.R.; Garibaldi, R.A.; Wilfert, J.N. and Smith, C.B.: In vitro activity of tobramycin and gentamicin. Antimicrobial Agents and Chemotherapy 2: 236-241 (1972).

Brummett, R.E.; Hines, D.; Saine, B. and Vernon, J.: A comparative study of the ototoxicity of tobramycin and gentamicin. Archives of Otolaryngology 96: 505-512 (1972).

Bunn, P.A.: Kanamycin. Medical Clinics of North America 54: 1245-1256 (1970).

Cabana, B.E. and Taggart, J.G.: Comparative pharmacokinetics of BB-K8 and kanamycin in dogs and humans. Antimicrobial Agents and Chemotherapy 3: 478-483 (1973).

Christensen, E.W.; Herrell, W.E. and Gilboy, J.T.: The effect of dihydrodesoxy streptomycin on the function of the eighth nerve; in Antibiotics Annual, p.552-555 (Antibiotica Inc., New York 1960).

Cox, C.E.: Gentamicin. A new aminoglycoside antibiotic. Clinical and laboratory studies in urinary tract infection. Journal of Infectious Diseases *119:* 486-491 (1969).

Crofton, J.W. and Douglas, A.S.: in Respiratory Diseases (Blackwell, Oxford 1969).

Crowe, C.C. and Sanders, E.: Is there complete cross-resistance of Gram-negative bacilli to gentamicin and tobramycin. Antimicrobial Agents and Chemotherapy *2:* 415-416 (1972).

Cutler, R.E.; Gulselynck, M.; Fleet, W.P. and Forrey, A.W.: Correlation of serum creatinine and gentamicin half life. Journal of the American Medical Association *219:* 1037-1041 (1972).

Cutler, R.E. and Orme, B.M.: Correlation of serum creatinine concentration and kanamycin half life. Journal of the American Medical Association *209:* 539-542 (1969).

Dans, P.E.; Barrett, F.F.; Casey, J.I. and Finland, M.: Klebsiella-Enterobacter in Boston City Hospital. Arch. intern. Med. *125:* 94-101 (1970).

Del Bene, V.E. and Farrar, W.E.: Tobramycin: *In vitro* activity and comparison with kanamycin and gentamicin. Antimicrobial Agents and Chemotherapy *1:* 340-342 (1972).

Dienstag, J. and Neu, H.C.: *In vitro* studies of tobramycin, an aminoglycoside antibiotic. Antimicrobial Agents and Chemotherapy *1:* 41-45 (1972).

Drasar, F.A.; Farrell, W.; Maskell, J. and Williams, J.D.: Tobramycin, amikacin, sissomicin, and gentamicin gram-negative rods. British Medical Journal *2:* 1284-1287 (1976).

Dye, W.E.: Bacteriology of tuberculosis with special reference to kanamycin and related drugs. Annals of the New York Academy of Sciences *132:* 901-904 (1966).

Emond, R.T.D.; Gray, J.A.; Smith, H. and Young, S.E.J.: Antibiotics in acute gastroenteritis. Lancet *1:* 312 (1969).

Ervin, F.R.; Bullock, W.E. and Nuttall, C.E.: Inactivation of gentamicin by penicillins in patients with renal failure. Antimicrobial Agents and Chemotherapy *9:* 1004-1011 (1976).

Falco, F.G.; Millard-Smith, H. and Arcieri, G.M.: Nephrotoxicity of aminoglycosides and gentamicin. Journal of Infectious Diseases *119:* 406-409 (1969).

Feathers, R.S.; Lewis, A.A.M.; Sagor, G.R.; Amirak, I.D. and Noone, P.: Prophylactic systemic antibiotics in colorectal surgery. Lancet *2:* 4-8 (1977).

Feld, R.; Valdivieso, M.; Bodey, G.P. and Rodriguez, V.: Comparison of amikacin and tobramycin in the treatment of infection in patients with cancer. Journal of Infectious Diseases *135:* 61-66 (1977).

Finegold, S.M.: Toxicity of kanamycin in adults. Ann. NY Acad. Sci. *132:* 942-956 (1966).

Fujii, R.: Patterns of organisms in disease and 'in vitro' sensitivity to kanamycin in comparison with other antibiotics. Annals of the New York Academy of Sciences *132:* 776-793 (1966).

Geddes, A.M.; Goodall, J.A.D.; Speirs, C.F.; Gillett, A.P.; Andrews, J. and Williams, J.D.: Clinical and laboratory studies with tobramycin. Chemotherapy (Basel) *20:* 245-256 (1974).

Gingell, J.C. and Waterworth, P.M.: Dose of gentamicin in patients with normal renal function and renal impairment. British Medical Journal *2:* 19-22 (1968).

Gordon, R.C.; Regamey, C. and Kirby, W.M.M.: Serum protein binding of the aminoglycoside antibiotics. Antimicrobial Agents and Chemotherapy *2:* 214-216 (1972).

Gray, J.; McGhie, D. and Ball, A.P.: Serratia marcescens: Antibacterial susceptibility and synergy. In Current Chemotherapy p.434. (American Society for Microbiology, Washington D.C., 1978).

Hahn, F.E. and Sarre, S.G.: Mechanism of action of gentamicin. Journal of Infectious Diseases *119:* 364-369 (1969).

Healy, J.C.; Drum, P.J. and Elliott, A.J.: Kanamycin dosage in renal failure. Australian and New Zealand Journal of Medicine *3:* 474-479 (1973).

Hoff, G.E.; Schiotz, P.O. and Paulsen, J.: Tobramycin treatment of *Pseudomonas aeruginosa* infections in cystic fibrosis. Scandinavian Journal of Infectious Diseases *6:* 333-337 (1974).

Howard, J.B. and McCracken, G.H.: Pharmacological evaluation of amikacin in neonates. Antimicrobial Agents and Chemotherapy *8:* 86-90 (1975).

Howard, J.B.; McCracken, G.H.; Trujillo, H. and Mohs, E.: Amikacin in newborn infants: comparative pharmacology with kanamycin and clinical efficacy in 45 neonates with bacterial diseases. Antimicrobial Agents and Chemotherapy *10:* 205-210 (1976).

Jackson, G.G.: Gentamicin. Practitioner *198:* 855-866 (1967).

Jackson, G.G. and Arcieri, G.: Ototoxicity of gentamicin in man. A survey and controlled analysis of clinical experience in the US Journal of Infectious Diseases *124* (Suppl. Dec): 130-137 (1971).

Kabins, S.A.; Nathan, G.R. and Cohen, S.: R-factor mediated resistance to gentamicin in a clinical isolate of *E. coli.* Journal of Infectious Diseases *124* (Suppl. Dec): 65-67 (1971).

Kabins, S.A.; Nathan, C. and Cohen, S.: *In vitro* comparison of netilmicin, a semisynthetic derivative of sisomicin, and four other aminoglycoside antibiotics. Antimicrobial Agents and Chemotherapy *10:* 139-145 (1976).

Kaneko, Y.; Nakagawa, T. and Tanaka, K.: Reissner's membrane after kanamycin administration. Archives of Otolaryngology *92:* 457-462 (1970).

Kaplan, J.M.; McCracken, G.H.; Thomas, M.L.; Horton, L.J. and Davis, N.: Clinical pharmacology of tobramycin in newborns. American Journal of Diseases of the Child *125:* 656-660 (1973).

Kass, I.: Kanamycin in the therapy of pulmonary tuberculosis in the United States. Annals of the New York Academy of Sciences *132:* 942-956 (1966).

Keusch, G.T.; Troncale, F.J. and Buchanan, R.D.: Malabsorption due to paromomycin. Archives of Internal Medicine *125:* 273-276 (1970).

Kucers, A.: in The Use of Antibiotics, p.157 (Heinemann, London 1972).

Kunin, C.M.: Absorption, distribution, excretion and fate of kanamycin. Annals of the New York Academy of Sciences *132:* 811-818 (1966).

Kunin, C.M.: A guide to use of antibiotics in patients with renal disease. Annals of Internal Medicine *67:* 151-158 (1967).

Kunin, C.M.; Chalmers, T.C.; Leevy, C.M.; Sebastyen, S.C.; Lieber, C.S. and Finland, M.: Absorption of orally administered neomycin and kanamycin with special reference to patients with severe hepatitis and renal disease. New England Journal of Medicine *262:* 380-385 (1960).

Kunin, C.M. and Finland, M.: Restrictions imposed on antibiotic therapy by renal failure. Archives of Internal Medicine *104:* 1030-1050 (1959).

Last, P.M. and Sherlock, S.: Systemic absorption of orally administered neomycin in liver disease. New England Journal of Medicine *262:* 385-387 (1960).

Leading Article: Staphylococci resistant to neomycin and bacitracin. Lancet *2:* 421-422 (1965).

Leading Article: Deafness after topical neomycin. British Medical Journal *4:* 181-182 (1969).

Levy, R.I. and Rifkind, B.M.: Lipid lowering drugs and hyperlipidaemia. Drugs *6:* 12 (1973).

Lockwood, W.R. and Bower, J.D.: Tobramycin and gentamicin concentrations in the serum of normal and anephric patients. Antimicrobial Agents and Chemotherapy *3:* 125-129 (1973).

Luft, F.C.; Yum, M.N. and Kleit, S.A.: Comparative nephrotoxicities of gentamicin and netilmicin in rats. Antimicrobial Agents and Chemotherapy *10:* 845-849 (1976).

McCracken, G.H.; Chrane, D.F. and Thomas, M.L.: Pharmacologic evaluation of gentamicin in newborn infants. Journal of Infectious Diseases *124* (Suppl. Dec): 214-223 (1971).

McLaughlin, J.E. and Reeves, D.S.: Clinical and laboratory evidence for inactivation of gentamicin by carbenicillin. Lancet *1:* 261-264 (1971).

McMillan, B.G.: Gentamicin in management of thermal injuries. Journal of Infectious Diseases *119:* 492-503 (1969).

Martin, C.M.; Ikari, N.S.; Zimmerman, J. and Waitz, J.A.: A virulent nosocomial Klebsiella with transferable R-factor for gentamicin. Emergence and Suppression. Journal of Infectious Diseases *124* (Suppl. Dec): 24-29 (1971).

Martin, C.M.; Cuomo, A.J.; Geraghty, M.J.; Zager, J.R. and Mandes, T.C.: Gram-negative rod bacteraemia. Journal of Infectious Diseases *119:* 506-517 (1969).

Martin, W.J.: The present status of streptomycin in antimicrobial therapy. Medical Clinics of North America *54*: 1161-1172 (1970).

Mawer, G.E.; Lucas, S.B. and McGough, J.G.: Nomogram for kanamycin dosage. Lancet *2*: 45 (1972).

Meyer, R.D.; Lewis, R.P.; Carmalt, E.D. and Finegold, S.M.: Amikacin therapy for serious gram-negative bacillary infections. Annals of Internal Medicine *83*: 790-800 (1975).

Meyer, R.D.; Halter, J.; Lewis, R.P. and White, M.: Gentamicin-resistant *Pseudomonas aeruginosa* and *Serratia marcescens* in a general hospital. Lancet *1*: 580-583 (1976a).

Meyers, B.R.; Hirschman, S.Z.; Yancovitz, S. and Ribner, B.: Pharmacokinetic parameters of sisomicin. Antimicrobial Agents and Chemotherapy *10*: 25-27 (1976b).

Miller, G.H.; Arcieri, G.; Weinstein, M.J. and Waitz, J.A.: Biological activity of netilmicin, a broad-spectrum semisynthetic aminoglycoside antibiotic. Antimicrobial Agents and Chemotherapy *10*: 827-836 (1976).

Morrice McCrae, W.M.; Raeburn, J.A. and Hanson, E.J.: Tobramycin therapy of infections due to *Pseudomonas aeruginosa* in patients with cystic fibrosis: effect of dosage and concentration of antibiotic in sputum. Journal of Infectious Diseases *134* (Suppl.): S191-193 (1976).

Murdoch, J. McC.; Gray, J.A.; Geddes, A.M. and Wallace, E.T.: Clinical experiences with kanamycin in septicaemia caused by Gram-negative organisms. Annals of New York Academy of Sciences *132*: 842-849 (1966).

Naber, K.G.; Westenfelder, S.R. and Madsen, P.O.: Pharmacokinetics of the aminoglycoside antibiotic tobramycin in humans. Antimicrobial Agents and Chemotherapy *3*: 469-473 (1973).

Neu, H.C. and Bendush, C.L.: Ototoxicity of tobramycin: a clinical overview. Journal of Infectious Diseases *134* (Suppl.): S206-218 (1976).

Newman, R.L. and Holt, R.J.: Gentamicin in paediatrics. Report on intrathecal gentamicin. Journal of Infectious Diseases *124* (Suppl. Dec): 254-256 (1971).

Noone, P.; Parsons, T.M.C.; Pattison, J.R.; Slack, R.C.B.; Garfield-Davies, D. and Hughes, K.: Experience in monitoring gentamicin therapy during treatment of serious Gram-negative sepsis. British Medical Journal *1*: 477-481 (1974a).

Noone, P.; Pattison, J.R. and Garfield-Davies, D.: The effective use of gentamicin in life threatening sepsis. Postgraduate Medical Journal *50* (Suppl. 7): 9-16 (1974b).

Noone, P. and Pattison, J.R.: Therapeutic implications of interaction of gentamicin and penicillins. Lancet *2*: 575-578 (1971).

Nyhan, W.L.: Toxicity of drugs in the newborn. Journal of Pediatrics *59*: 1-20 (1961).

Pechere, J-C.; Pechere, M-M. and Dugal, R.: Clinical pharmacokinetics of sisomicin: dosage schedules in renal-impaired patients. Antimicrobial Agents and Chemotherapy *9*: 761-765 (1976).

Pennington, J.E.; Dale, D.C.; Reynolds, H.Y. and MacLowry, J.D.: Gentamicin sulfate pharmacokinetics: lower levels of gentamicin in blood during fever. Journal of Infectious Diseases *132*: 270-275 (1975).

Petersdorf, R.G. and Turck, M.: Kanamycin in urinary tract infections. Annals of the New York Academy of Sciences *132*: 834-841 (1966).

Reynolds, A.V.; Hamilton-Miller, J.M.T. and Brumfitt, W.: Newer aminoglycosides — amikacin and tobramycin: an in-vitro comparison with kanamycin and gentamicin. British Medical Journal *3*: 778-780 (1974).

Riff, L.J. and Jackson, G.G.: Pharmacology of gentamicin in man. Journal of Infectious Diseases *124* (Suppl. Dec): 98-104 (1971).

Riff, L.J. and Jackson, G.G.: Laboratory and clinical conditions for gentamicin inactivation by carbenicillin. Archives of Internal Medicine *130*: 887-891 (1972).

Sabath, L.D.: Current concepts. Drug resistance of bacteria. New England Journal of Medicine *280*: 91-94 (1969).

Sande, M.A. and Irvin, R.G.: Penicillin-aminoglycoside synergy in experimental *Streptococcus viridans* endocarditis. Journal of Infectious Diseases *129*: 572-576 (1974).

Schnurr. L.P.; Ball, A.P.; Geddes, A.M.; Gray, J. and McGhie, D.: Bacterial endocarditis in England in the 1970's. Quarterly Journal of Medicine *46*: 499-512 (1977).

Shulman. J.A.; Terry, P.M. and Hough. C.E.: Colonization with gentamicin resistant *Pseudomonas aeruginosa*, pyocine type 5 in a burn unit. Journal of Infectious Diseases *124* (Suppl. Dec): 18-23 (1971).

Simon, H.J.: Streptomycin, kanamycin, neomycin and paromomycin. Paediatric Clinics of North America *15*: 73-83 (1968).

Simon, H.J. and Axline, S.G.: Clinical pharmacology of kanamycin in premature infants. Annals of the New York Academy of Sciences *132*: 1020-1025 (1966).

Simon, V.K.; Mosinger, E.U. and Malerczy, V.: Pharmacokinetic studies of tobramycin and gentamicin. Antimicrobial Agents and Chemotherapy *3*: 445-450 (1973).

Snelling, C.F.T.; Ronald, A.R.; Cates, C.Y. and Forsythe, W.C.: Resistance of Gram-negative bacilli to gentamicin. Journal of Infectious Diseases *124* (Suppl. Dec): 264-270 (1971).

Stratford, B.C.; Dixson, S. and Cobcroft, A.J.: Serum levels of gentamicin and tobramycin after slow intravenous bolus injection. Lancet *1*: 378-379 (1974).

Tally, F.P.; Louie. T.J.; Weinstein. W.M.; Bartlett, J.G. and Gorbach, S.L.: Amikacin therapy for severe gram-negative sepsis: emphasis on infections with gentamicin-resistant organisms. Annals of Internal Medicine *83*: 484-488 (1975).

Today's Drugs: Lipid lowering agents. British Medical Journal *2*: 643 (1972).

Trimble, G.X.: Neomycin ototoxicity: Dossier and Doses. New England Journal of Medicine *281*: 219 (1969).

Waitz, J.A.; Moss, E.L.; Drube, C.G. and Weinstein, M.J.: Comparative activity of sisomycin, gentamicin, kanamycin and tobramycin. Antimicrobial Agents and Chemotherapy *2*: 431-437 (1972).

Waitz, J.A. and Weinstein, M.J.: Recent microbiological studies with gentamicin. Journal of Infectious Diseases *119*: 355-360 (1969).

Watanakunakorn, C.: Penicillin combined with gentamicin or streptomycin: synergism against *Enterococci*. Journal of Infectious Diseases *124*: 581-586 (1971).

Waterworth, P.M.: The *in vitro* activity of tobramycin compared with that of other aminoglycosides. Journal of Clinical Pathology *25*: 979-983 (1972).

Wersall, J.; Lundquist, R.G. and Bjorkroth, B.: Ototoxicity of gentamicin. Journal of Infectious Diseases *119*: 410-415 (1969).

Wick, W.E. and Welles, J.S.: Nebramycin. A new broad spectrum antibiotic complex. IV. *In vitro* and *in vivo* laboratory evaluation. Antimicrobial Agents and Chemotherapy, p.341-348 (1967).

Wilson, P. and Ramsden, R.T.: Immediate effects of tobramycin on human cochlea and correlation with serum tobramycin levels. British Medical Journal *1*: 259-261 (1977).

Winters, R.E.; Chow, A.W.; Hecht, R.H. and Hewitt, W.L.: Combined use of gentamicin and carbenicillin. Annals of Internal Medicine *75*: 925-927 (1971).

16. Metronidazole

Busch, D.F.; Sutter, V.L. and Finegold, S.M.: Activity of combinations of antibacterial agents against Bacteroides fragilis. Journal of Infectious Diseases *133*: 321-328 (1976).

Davies, A.H.: Metronidazole in human infections with syphilis. British Journal of Venereal Diseases *43*: 197-200 (1967).

Eykyn, S.J. and Phillips, I.: Metronidazole and anaerobic sepsis. British Medical Journal *2*: 1418-1421 (1976).

Finegold, S.M.; Bartlett, A.W., Chow, D.J. et al.: Management of anaerobic infections. Annals of Internal Medicine *83*: 375-389 (1975).

Gray, M.S.; Kane, P.O. and Squires, S.: Further observations on metronidazole (Flagyl). British Journal of Venereal Diseases *37*: 278-279 (1961).

Hamilton-Miller, J.M.T.: Antimicrobial agents acting against anaerobes. Journal of Antimicrobial Chemotherapy *1*: 273-289 (1975).

Ingham, H.R.; Selkon, J.B. and Hale, J.H.: The antibacterial activity of metronidazole. Journal of Antimicrobial Chemotherapy *1*: 355-361 (1975a).

Ingham, H.R.; Selkon, J.B. and Hale, J.H.: Treatment with metronidazole of three patients with serious infections due to Bacteroides fragilis. Journal of Antimicrobial Chemotherapy *1*: 235-242 (1975b).

Nastro, L.J. and Finegold, S.M.: Bactericidal activity of five antimicrobial agents against Bacteroides fragilis. Journal of Infectious Diseases *126*: 104-107 (1972).

Salem, A.R.; Jackson, D.D. and McFadzean, J.A.: An investigation of interactions between metronidazole (Flagyl) and other antibacterial agents. Journal of Antimicrobial Chemotherapy *1*: 382-391 (1975).

Selkon, J.B.; Hale, J.H. and Ingham, H.R.: Metronidazole in the treatment of anaerobic infection in man. Proceedings of the 9th International Congress of Chemotherapy (London 1975).

Shinn, D.L.S.: Metronidazole in acute ulcerative gingivitis. Lancet *1*: 1191 (1962).

Study Group: An evaluation of metronidazole in the prophylaxis and treatment of anaerobic infections in surgical patients. Journal of Antimicrobial Chemotherapy *1*: 393-401 (1975).

Tally, F.P.; Sutter, V.L. and Finegold, S.M.: Treatment of anaerobic infections with metronidazole. Antimicrobial Agents and Chemotherapy *7*: 672-675 (1975).

Welling, P.G. and Monro, A.M.: The pharmacokinetics of metronidazole and tinidazole in man. Arzneimittel-Forschung *22*: 2128-2132 (1972).

Willis, A.T. et al.: Metronidazole in prevention and treatment of Bacteroides infections after appendicectomy. British Medical Journal *1*: 318-321 (1976).

Willis, A.T. et al.: Metronidazole in prevention and treatment of Bacteroides infections in elective colonic surgery. British Medical Journal *1*: 607-610 (1977).

17. Antituberculosis Drugs

Fox, W.: Realistic chemotherapeutic policies for tuberculosis in the developing countries. British Medical Journal *1*: 135 (1964).

Fox, W.: General considerations in the choice and management of regimens of chemotherapy for pulmonary tuberculosis. Bull. Un. int. Tuberc. *47*: 30 (1972).

Ross, J.D. and Horne, N.W.: Modern Drug Treatment in Tuberculosis 5th Ed. (The Chest, Heart and Stroke Association) Health Horizon, London (1976).

18. Chemotherapy of Gram-negative Bacillary Infections

Aserkoff, B. and Bennett, J.V.: Effect of antibiotic therapy in acute salmonellosis on the fecal excretion of salmonellae. New England Journal of Medicine *281*: 636-640 (1969).

Ball, A.P.; McGhie, D. and Geddes, A.M.: Serratia marcescens in a general hospital. Quarterly Journal of Medicine *46*: 63-71 (1977).

Christie, A.B.: Treatment of typhoid carriers with ampicillin. British Medical Journal *1*: 1609-1611 (1964).

Christie, A.B.: Treatment of Gastrointestinal Infections; in Geddes and Williams (Eds) A Clinician's Viewpoint in Current Antibiotic Therapy, Chapter 17, p.183-193 (Churchill Livingstone, Edinburgh and London 1973).

Davies, J.R.; Farrant, W.N. and Uttley, A.H.C.: Antibiotic resistance of *Shigella sonnei*. Lancet *2*: 1157-1159 (1970).

Felty, A.R. and Keefer, C.S.: *Bacillus coli* sepsis: a clinical study of 28 cases of blood stream infection by the colon bacillus. Journal of the American Medical Association *82*: 1430-1433 (1924).

Finland, M.; Jones, W.F. and Barnes, M.W.: Occurrence of serious bacterial infections since the introduction of antibacterial agents. Journal of the American Medical Association *170*: 2188-2197 (1959).

Geddes, A.M.: The antibiotic treatment of typhoid fever. Journal of Antimicrobial Chemotherapy *3*: 382-383 (1977).

Geddes, A.M.; Fothergill, R.; Goodall, J.A.D. and Dorken, P.R.: Evaluation of trimethoprim — sulphamethoxazole compound in treatment of Salmonella infections. British Medical Journal *3*: 451-454 (1971).

Geddes, A.M. and Goodall, J.A.D.: Chloramphenicol resistance in the typhoid bacillus. British Medical Journal *3*: 525 (1972).

Gillies, R.R.: Treatment of gastrointestinal infection; in Geddes and Williams (Eds) A bacteriologist's viewpoint in current antibiotic therapy, Chapter 16, p.177-182 (Churchill Livingstone, Edinburgh and London 1973).

Gray, J.A.; Geddes, A.M.; Wallace, E.T. and Murdoch, J. McC.: The long-term management of urinary infections with cycloserine. British Journal of Urology (Suppl). Symposium on Pyelonephritis. p.33-38 (1967).

Greene, W.H.; Moody, M.; Schimpff, S.; Young, V.M. and Wiernik, P.H.: *Pseudomonas aeruginosa* resistant to carbenicillin and gentamicin. Epidemiologic and clinical aspects in a cancer center. Annals of Internal Medicine *79*: 684-689 (1973).

Hall, W.H. and Gold, D.: Shock associated with bacteremia. Archives of Internal Medicine *96*: 403-412 (1955).

Herrell, W.E. and Brown, A.E.: The treatment of septicemia: results before and after the advent of sulfamido compounds. Journal of the American Medical Association *116*: 179-183 (1941).

Johnston, R.N.; McNeil, R.S.; Smith, D.H.; Dempster, M.B.; Nairn, J.R.; Purvis, M.S.; Watson, J.M. and Ward, F.G.: Five year winter chemoprophylaxis for chronic bronchitis. British Medical Journal *4*: 265-269 (1969).

Joint Project by Members of the Association for the Study of Infectious Diseases: Effect of neomycin in non-invasive salmonella infections of the gastrointestinal tract. Lancet *2*: 1159-1161 (1970).

Jonsson, M.: Pivmecillinam in the treatment of salmonella carriers. Journal of Antimicrobial Chemotherapy *3 (Suppl. B)*: 103-107 (1977).

Lancet: Septic Shock (Annotation) *2*: 1265-1266 (1963).

Leading Article: Salmonella typhi resistant to chloramphenicol. British Medical Journal *3*: 306-307 (1972).

Leading Article: Chloramphenicol Resistance in Typhoid. Lancet *2*: 1008-1009 (1973).

McAllister, T.A.: Urinary tract infections in Scottish rural general practice: A postal study using dipslides. Journal of International Medical Research *2*: 400-408 (1974).

McCabe, W.R. and Jackson, G.G.: Gram-negative bacteremia. I. Etiology and ecology. II. Clinical, laboratory and therapeutic observations. Archives of Internal Medicine *110*: 847-855, 856-864 (1962).

McCracken, G.H. and Shinefield, H.R.: Changes in the pattern of neonatal septicaemia and meningitis. American Journal of Diseases of Childhood *112*: 33-39 (1966).

Maiztegui, J.I.; Biegeleisen, J.Z.; Cherry, W.B. and Kass, E.H.: Bacteremia due to gram-negative rods. A clinical, bacteriologic, serologic and immunofluorescent study. New England Journal of Medicine *272*: 222-229 (1965).

Malone, D.N.; Gould, J.C. and Grant, I.W.B.: A comparative study of ampicillin, tetracycline and methacycline in acute exacerbation of chronic bronchitis. Lancet *2*: 594-596 (1968).

Martin, W.J. and McHenry, M.C.: 59 cases of bacteremic shock due to gram-negative enteric bacilli. Medical Clinics of North America *46*: 1073-1097 (1962).

MRC Working Party: Value of chemoprophylaxis and chemotherapy in early chronic bronchitis. British Medical Journal *1*: 117-122 (1966).

Murdoch, J. McC.; Geddes, A.M.; Tulloch, W.S.; Newsam, J.E.; Thomson, W.N.; Bidwell, D. and

Wallace, E.T.: The problem of pyelonephritis: a four year study of a pyelonephritis unit. Practitioner *196*: 800-810 (1966a).

Murdoch, J. McC.; Gray, J.A.; Geddes, A.M. and Wallace, E.T.: Clinical experiences with kanamycin in septicemia caused by Gram-negative organisms. Annals of the New York Academy of Sciences *132*: 842-849 (1966b).

Murdoch, J. McC.; Sleigh, J.D. and Frazer, S.C.: Cycloserine in treatment of infection of urinary tract. British Medical Journal *2*: 1055-1058 (1959).

Ormonde, N.W.H.; Gray, J.A.; Murdoch, J. McC.; Wallace, E.T.; Brumfitt, W.; Pursell, R. and Regan, J.W.: Chronic bacteriuria due to *Escherichia coli* I Assessment of the value of combined short- and long-term treatment with cycloserine, nitrofurantoin and sulphadimidine. Journal of Infectious Diseases *120*: 82-86 (1969).

Roe, E. and Lowbury, E.J.L.: Changes in antibiotic sensitivity patterns of Gram-negative bacilli in burns. Journal of Clinical Pathology *25*: 176-178 (1972).

Sabath, L.D.: Current concepts: Drug resistance of bacteria. New England Journal of Medicine *280*: 91-94 (1969).

Sardesai, H.V.; Karandikar, R.S. and Harshe, R.G.: Comparative trial of co-trimoxazole and chloramphenicol in typhoid fever. British Medical Journal *1*: 82-83 (1973).

Sharp, P.M.; Saenz, C.A. and Martin, R.R.: Amikacin (BB-K8) treatment of multiple-drug-resistant proteus infections. Antimicrobial Agents and Chemotherapy *5*: 435-438 (1974).

Shulman, J.A.; Terry, P.M. and Hough, C.E.: Colonization with gentamicin-resistant Pseudomonas aeruginosa, pyocine type 5, in a burn unit. Journal of Infectious Diseases *124*: (Suppl.): 18-23 (1971).

Spittel, J.A.; Martin, W.J. and Nichols, D.R.: Bacteremia owing to Gram-negative bacilli: experiences in the treatment of 137 patients in a 15 year period. Annals of Internal Medicine *44*: 302-315 (1956).

Weil, M.H.; Shubin, H. and Biddle, M.: Shock caused by Gram-negative micro-organisms. Analysis of 169 cases. Annals of Internal Medicine *60*: 384-400 (1964).

Weil, M.H. and Spink, W.W.: The shock syndrome associated with bacteremia due to Gram-negative bacilli. Archives of Internal Medicine *101*: 184-193 (1958).

Williams, G.T.; Houang, E.T.; Shaw, E.J.; Tobaqchali, S.: Bacteraemia in a London teaching hospital 1966-75. Lancet *2*: 1291-1293 (1976).

20. Antibacterial Therapy in Renal and Hepatic Disease

Bhagwat, A.G. and Warren, R.E.: Hepatic reaction to nitrofurantoin. Lancet *2*: 1369 (1969).

Bulger, R.J.; Lindholm, D.D.; Murray, J.S. and Kirby, W.M.M.: Effect of uremia on methicillin and oxacillin blood levels. Journal of the American Medical Association *187*: 319-322 (1964).

Conn, H.O.; Binder, H.J. and Orr, H.D.: Ethionamide-induced hepatitis: a review with a report on an additional case. American Review of Respiratory Diseases *90*: 542-552 (1964).

Curtis, J.R. and Eastwood, J.B.: Colistin sulphomethate sodium administration in the presence of severe renal failure and during haemodialysis and peritoneal dialysis. British Medical Journal *1*: 484-485 (1968).

Dismukes, W.E.: Oxacillin-induced hepatic dysfunction. Journal of the American Medical Association *226*: 861-863 (1973).

Dujovne, C.A.; Chan, C.H. and Zimmerman, H.J.: Sulphonamide hepatic injury. New England Journal of Medicine *277*: 785-788 (1967).

Eastwood, J.B. and Curtis, J.R.: Carbenicillin administration in patients with severe renal failure. British Medical Journal *1*: 486-487 (1968).

Fischer, E.: Renal excretion of sulphadimidine in normal and uraemic subjects. Lancet *2*: 210-212 (1972).

Garrod, L.P.; Lambert, H.P. and O'Grady, F.: in Dosage in Antibiotic and Chemotherapy 4th Ed, Chapter 17, p.291-306 (Churchill Livingstone, Edinburgh and London 1973).

Gray, J.A.; Geddes, A.M.; Wallace, E.T. and Murdoch, J. McC.: Symposium on Pyelonephritis, Edinburgh 1966. Supplement to British Journal of Urology, p.33-37 (E and S Livingstone, Edinburgh 1967).

Hoeprich, P.R.: The polymyxins. Medical Clinics of North America 54: 1257-1265 (1970).

Knirsch, A.K. and Gralla, E.J.: Serum transaminase levels after parenteral ampicillin and carbenicillin administration. New England Journal of Medicine 282: 1081-1082 (1970).

Kovnat, P.; Labovitz, E. and Levison, S.P.: Antibiotics and the kidney. Medical Clinics of North America 57: 1045-1063 (1973).

Kucers, A. and Bennett, N. McK.: in Lincomycin and Clindamycin in the Use of Antibiotics 2nd Ed p.284-302 (William Heinemann Medical Books, London 1975).

Kunin, C.M.: A guide to the use of antibiotics in patients with renal disease. Annals of Internal Medicine 67: 151-158 (1967).

Kunin, C.M.; Glazko, A.J. and Finland, M.: Persistence of antibiotics in blood of patients with acute renal failure. II Chloramphenicol and its metabolic products in the blood of patients with severe renal disease or hepatic cirrhosis. Journal of Clinical Investigations 38: 1498-1508 (1959).

Leading Article: Tetracycline and blood urea. British Medical Journal 3: 370 (1972).

Lepper, M.H.; Wolfe, C.K.; Zimmerman, H.J.; Caldwell, E.R.; Spies, H.W. and Dowling, H.F.: Effect of large doses of aureomycin on human liver. Archives of Internal Medicine 88: 271-283 (1951).

Lew, H.T. and French, S.W.: Tetracycline nephrotoxicity and nonoliguric acute renal failure. Archives of Internal Medicine 118: 123-128 (1966).

McGeachie, J.; Girdwood, R.W.A.; Burton, J.A. and Kennedy, A.C.: Impaired renal function and serum levels of rifamide. Scottish Medical Journal 15: 257-260 (1970).

Moulding, T.S. and Goldstein, S.: Hepatotoxicity due to ethionamide. American Review of Respiratory Diseases 86: 252-255 (1962).

Ogg, C.S.; Toseland, P.A. and Cameron, J.S.: Pulmonary tuberculosis in patients on intermittent haemodialysis. British Medical Journal 2: 283-284 (1968).

O'Grady, F.: Antibiotics in renal failure. British Medical Bulletin 27: 142-147 (1971).

Phillips, S. and Tashman, H.: Ethionamide jaundice. American Review of Respiratory Diseases 87: 896-898 (1963).

Plaut, M.E.; O'Connell, C.J.; Pabico, R.C. and Davidson, D.: Penicillin handling in normal and azotemic patients. Journal of Laboratory and Clinical Medicine 74: 12-18 (1969).

Schultz, J.C.; Adamson, J.S.; Workman, W.W. and Norman, T.W.: Fatal liver disease after intravenous administration of tetracycline in high dosage. New England Journal of Medicine 269: 999-1004 (1963).

Strauss, W. and Jawetz, E.: Nitrofurantoin in patients with hepatic dysfunction. Clinical Pharmacology and Therapeutics 4: 297-303 (1963).

Welling, P.G.; Craig, W.A.; Amidon, G.L. and Kunin, C.M.: Pharmacokinetics of trimethoprim and sulfamethoxazole in normal subjects and in patients with renal failure. Journal of Infectious Diseases 128 (Suppl.): 556-566 (1973).

21. Antibacterial Therapy in Infants and Children

Alder, V.G.; Burman, D.; Corner, B.D. and Gillespie, W.A.: Absorption of hexachlorophene from infant's skin. Lancet 2: 384-385 (1972).

Altemeier, W.A. and Ayoub, E.M.: Erythromycin prophylaxis for pertussis. Pediatrics 59: 623-625 (1977).

Anderson, E.: Childhood complications of nalidixic acid. Journal of the American Medical Association 216: 1023-1024 (1971).

Axline, S.G.; Yaffe, S.J. and Simon, H.J.: Clinical pharmacology of antimicrobials in premature infants: II Ampicillin, methicillin, oxacillin, neomycin and colistin. Pediatrics 39: 97-107 (1967).

Barnett, H.L.; McNamara, H.; Shultz, S. and Tompsett, R.: Renal clearances of sodium penicillin G, pro-
    caine penicillin G and insulin in infants and children. Pediatrics 3: 418-422 (1949).
Burland, W.L. and Simpson, K.: Administration of cephaloridine to the newborn infant. Postgraduate
    Medical Journal 43: (Suppl.): 112-115 (1967).
Burns, L. and Hodgman, J.: Studies of prematures given erythromycin estolate. American Journal of
    Diseases of Children 106: 280-288 (1963).
Burns, L.E.; Hodgman, J.E. and Cass, A.B.: Fatal circulatory collapse in premature infants receiving
    chloramphenicol. New England Journal of Medicine 261: 1318-1321 (1959).
Burns, M.W. and May, J.R.: Bacterial precipitins in serum of patients with cystic fibrosis. Lancet 1:
    270-272 (1968).
Cocke, J.G.; Brown, R.E. and Geppert, L.J.: Optic neuritis with prolonged use of chloramphenicol. Jour-
    nal of Pediatrics 68: 27-31 (1966).
Cohlan, S.Q.; Bevelander, G. and Tiamsic, T.: Growth inhibition of prematures receiving tetracycline.
    American Journal of Diseases of Children 105: 453-461 (1963).
Dahnsjö, H., Andersson, H., Hallander, H.O. et al.: Tone audiometry control of children treated for
    meningitis with large intravenous doses of ampicillin. Acta Paediatrica Scandinavica, 65: 733-737
    (1976).
Davies, P.A.; Darrell, J.H.; Chandran, K.R. and Waterworth, P.M.: The efficacy of antibiotics in the
    neonatal period; in Watt (Ed) The Control of Chemotherapy, p.49-68 (E & S Livingstone, Edin-
    burgh and London 1970).
Finegold, S.M. and Ziment, I.: Sulfonamides, nitrofurans and nalidixic acid. Pediatric Clinics of North
    America 15: 95-105 (1968).
Garrod, L.P.; Lambert, H.P. and O'Grady, F.: in Dosage in Antibiotic and Chemotherapy 4th Ed Chapter
    17, p.291-306 (Churchill Livingstone, Edinburgh and London 1973a).
Garrod, L.P.; Lambert, H.P. and O'Grady, F.: in Sulphonamides in Antibiotic and Chemotherapy 4th Ed
    Chapter 2, p.12-28 (Churchill Livingstone, Edinburgh and London 1973b).
Garrod, L.P.; Lambert, H.P. and O'Grady, F.: in Meningitis in Antibiotic and Chemotherapy 4th Ed
    Chapter 20, p.347-361 (Churchill Livingstone, Edinburgh and London 1973c).
Gill, S. and Davis, J.A.: The pharmacology of the fetus, baby and growing child; in Davis and Dobbing
    (Eds) Scientific Foundations of Paediatrics, Chapter 45, p.801-818 (William Heinemann Medical
    Books, London 1974).
Heckmatt, J.Z.: Coliform meningitis in the newborn. Arch. Dis. Child. 51: 569-575 (1976).
Huang, N.N.; Robison, D.H.; Promadhattavedi, V. and Sproul, A.: Visual disturbances in cystic fibrosis
    following chloramphenicol administration. Journal of Pediatrics 68: 32-44 (1966).
Hutchison, J.H.: Some common disorders in infancy and early childhood; in Alstead and Girdwood (Eds)
    Textbook of Medical Treatment 13th Ed Chapter 23, p.528 (Churchill Livingstone, Edinburgh and
    London 1974).
Kaplan, J.M.; McCracken, G.H.; Horton, L.J.; Thomas, M.L. and Davis, N.: Pharmacologic studies in
    neonates given large doses of ampicillin. Journal of Pediatrics 84: 571-577 (1974).
Kucers, A. and Bennett, N. McK.: Sulphonamides in The Use of Antibiotics 2nd Ed p.432-451 (William
    Heinemann Medical Books, London 1975a).
Kucers, A. and Bennett, N. McK.: Tetracyclines in The Use of Antibiotics 2nd Ed p.381-416 (William
    Heinemann Medical Books, London, 1975b).
Kucers, A. and Bennett, N. McK.: Lincomycin and Clindamicin in the Use of Antibiotics 2nd Ed
    p.282-302 (William Heinemann Medical Books, London 1975c).
Kucers, A. and Bennett, N. McK.: Cephalothin and Cephaloridine in The Use of Antibiotics 2nd Ed
    p.126-145 (William Heinemann Medical Books, London 1975d).
Kunin, C.M.; Glazko, A.J. and Finland, M.: Persistence of antibiotics in blood of patients with acute renal
    failure. II Chloramphenicol and its metabolic products in the blood of patients with severe renal
    disease or hepatic cirrhosis. Journal of Clinical Investigation 38: 1498-1508 (1959).

Lambdin, M.A.; Waddell, W.W. and Birdsong, McL.: Chloramphenicol toxicity in the premature infant. Pediatrics *25*: 935-940 (1960).

Leach, R.H. and Wood, R.S.B.: Drug dosage for children. Lancet *2*: 1350-1351 (1967).

Liddy, N.: Intravenous fusidic acid in the newborn. Lancet *1*: 621 (1973). `

McCracken, G.H.; Ginsberg, C.; Chrane, D.F.; Thomas, M.L. and Horton, L.J.: Clinical pharmacology of penicillin in newborn infants. Journal of Pediatrics *82*: 692-698 (1973).

McCrae, W.M.: Management of cystic fibrosis, in Modern Trends in Paediatrics, 4th Ed. Chapter 6, p.157-179. Edited by John Apley. Butterworth, London (1974).

Marget, W.: Special aspects of cephalosporin therapy in infants and children. Postgraduate Medical Journal *47* (Suppl.): 54-57 (1971).

Mearns, M.B.: Cystic fibrosis. British Journal of Hospital Medicine *12*: 497-506 (1974).

Nelson, J.D. and McCracken, G.H.: Clinical pharmacology of carbenicillin and gentamicin in the neonate and comparative efficacy with ampicillin and gentamicin. Pediatrics *52*: 801-812 (1973).

Nyhan, W.L.: Toxicity of drugs in the neonate. Journal of Pediatrics *59*: 1-20 (1961).

Powell, H.; Swarner, O.; Gluck, L. and Lampert, P.: Hexachlorophene myelinopathy in premature infants. Journal of Pediatrics *82*: 976-981 (1973).

Raeburn, J.A.: Antibiotic management of cystic fibrosis. Journal of Antimicrobial Chemotherapy *2*: 107-108 (1976).

Riley, H.D.: The new penicillins and cephalosporins. Advances in Pediatrics *17*: 227-315 (1970).

Roy, L.P.: Sulphamethoxazole-Trimethoprim in infancy. Medical Journal of Australia *1*: 148-150 (1971).

Sparr, R.A. and Pritchard, J.A.: Maternal and newborn distribution and excretion of sulfamethoxypyridazine (Kynex). Obstetrics and Gynaecology *12*: 131-134 (1958).

Sutherland, J.M. and Keller, W.H.: Novobiocin and neonatal hyperbilirubinaemia. American Journal of Diseases of Children *101*: 447-453 (1961).

Thistlethwaite, D.: Pharmacology; in Cockburn and Drillien (Eds) Neonatal Medicine. Chapter 23, p. 752-787 (Blackwell Scientific Publication, Oxford, London, Edinburgh, Melbourne 1974).

Weiss, C.F.; Glazko, A.J. and Weston, J.K.: Chloramphenicol in the newborn infant: A physiologic explanation of its toxicity when given in excessive doses. New England Journal of Medicine *262*: 787-794 (1960).

Williams, R.F.: Colonization of the developing body by bacteria; in Davis and Dobbing (Eds) Scientific Foundations of Paediatrics. Chapter 44, p. 789-801 (William Heinemann Medical Books, London 1974).

Wise, R.I.: Modern management of Severe Staphylococcal Disease. Medicine *52*: 295-305 (1973).

Yaffe, S.J.: Antibiotic dosage in newborn and premature infants. Journal of the American Medical Association *193*: 818-820 (1965).

Yaffe, S.J. and Back, N.: Neonatal pharmacology. Pediatric Clinics of North America *13*: 527-541 (1966).

Yaffe, S.J. and Simon, H.J.: Clinical pharmacology of antibiotics in the neonate; in Watt (Ed) The Control of Chemotherapy, p.37-48 (E & S Livingstone, Edinburgh and London 1970).

23. Antibacterial Drugs in Obstetrics and Gynaecology

Murdoch, J. McC.: Urinary Tract Infection in the Female; in Keller (Ed) Modern Trends in Gynaecology, p.101-117 (Butterworths, London 1963).

25. Opportunistic Infections

Brumfitt, W.: Opportunistic Infections; in Jepson (Ed) Transactions of the Medical Society of London *88*: 102-109 (1972).

Freid, M.A. and Vosti, K.L.: The importance of underlying disease in patients with gram-negative bacteraemia. Archives of Internal Medicine *121:* 418 (1968).

Gould, J.C.: Bacterial Infections; in Finland, Marget and Bartmann (Eds) Opportunists and Opportunity in Infection p.71 (Springer-Verlag, Berlin, Heidelberg, New York 1971).

McCabe, W.R. and Jackson, G.G.: Gram-negative bacteremia. I aetiology and ecology. Archives of Internal Medicine *110:* 847 (1962a).

McCabe, W.R. and Jackson, G.G.: Gram-negative bacteremia. II clinical, laboratory and therapeutic observations. Archives of Internal Medicine *110:* 856 (1962b).

Murdoch, J. McC.; Speirs, C.F. and Pullen, H.: The bacteraemic shock syndrome. British Journal of Hospital Medicine *1:* 346 (1968).

Murdoch, J. McC.: Opportunistic Infections; in Jepson (Ed) Transactions of the Medical Society of London *88:* 109-115 (1972).

26. The Management of Tuberculosis

Seaton, A.: Diseases of the respiratory system: tuberculosis. British Medical Journal *1:* 701-703 (1978).

Subject Index